High-Intensity Strength Training

The Most Effective and Efficient Means for Developing Muscle and Strength

Wayne L. Westcott, Ph.D., CSCS
Tracy D'Arpino, B.S., LPTA

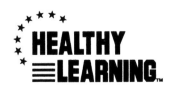

ISBN: 1-58518-724-0
Library of Congress Control Number: 2002112042
Cover design: Jennifer Bokelmann
Text design: Jeanne Hamilton
Front cover and author photos: ©Rosemary Tufankjian 2002
Text photos (pages 49 and 81): ©Rosemary Tufankjian 2002

Healthy Learning
P.O. Box 1828
Monterey, CA 93942
www.healthylearning.com

Dedication

We dedicate this book to the hundreds of participants in our high-intensity strength training research studies that we have conducted over the years, and to James Baker and J. Kelly Powell, who are in charge of physical fitness for the United States Navy.

Acknowledgments

We are privileged to acknowledge our professional colleagues and research participants, whose assistance and encouragement made this book possible. We first recognize our expert editorial team at *Healthy Learning*, Dr. Jim Peterson and Dr. Rick Frey. We are most grateful to Marsha Young, fitness administrative associate, for preparing the manuscript and providing editorial advice. Our special thanks to Olivia Chamberland, our outstanding cover model who has developed her award-winning physique through high-intensity training techniques, to Joe Thurston our other muscular model and five-time gold medallist at the International Police and Firefighter Combat Fighting Championship, as well as to Rosemary Tufankjian and Derik Rochon, our most talented photographers.

We also greatly appreciate the support of Claudia Westcott, Rita LaRosa Loud, Gayle Laing, Cindy Long, Adele Giurastante, Maureen Minihan, Bill Johnson, Mary Hurley, Ralph Yohe and all of the staff and members at the South Shore YMCA. Our indebtedness to Arthur Jones, Dr. Ellington Darden and Jim Teatum, all of whom have been associated with Nautilus in various capacities over the years. These individuals have played an instrumental role in developing and demonstrating the basic principles and techniques involved in high-intensity strength training. We are also most pleased with the interest and support that we have received from James Baker and J. Kelly Powell, who direct physical fitness for the United States Navy. Finally, we acknowledge God's grace in allowing us to research and write about these extremely safe, effective and efficient strength training procedures that we hope will enhance both your exercise sessions and your muscular development.

Table of Contents

Foreword

If you were to ask anyone in exercise science or the fitness industry who is the most credible and acknowledged strength expert in the field, the answer would most likely point to Dr. Wayne Westcott. Wayne is a phenomenal educator. This book is a tribute to his ability to present detailed and technical physiological data in a way that is practical, usable, and applicable to both personal trainers and fitness enthusiasts alike. *High-Intensity Strength Training* contains solid, pertinent, and current theoretical and practical information that thoroughly defines cutting-edge, strength-training techniques, along with in-depth progressive programming for each protocol. Wayne brings a unique quality of clarity and understanding to anything that he does. The comprehensive attention to every facet of training discussed in the book is thought-out and infused with Wayne's insightful and profound knowledge of strength-training principles, backed consistently by well-documented research data.

Wayne and his co-author, Tracy D'Arpino, have written an exceptionally complete and all-inclusive guide to advanced strength training. I have worked with Wayne for years; he is a mentor, a good friend, and someone whose work I truly respect.

Linda Shelton
Fitness Director
SHAPE Magazine

I

Introduction: Overview of High-Intensity Strength Training

High-intensity strength training is the most effective and efficient method for adding muscle and gaining strength, whether you are a fitness enthusiast or an advanced level athlete. Once you have cleared the initial exercise stage, you will find high-intensity strength training an excellent means for passing strength plateaus and attaining more muscularity. But before we explore the high-intensity training techniques, let's briefly review the recent history of strength exercise.

Prior to the 1970's, relatively few people performed strength exercise. Although weight training facilities could be found in some YMCAs and an occasional body building gym, the general public was essentially uninterested and uninvolved with this type of exercise. Most people at that time were firmly convinced that strength training was unnatural and unnecessary. The stereotypical image of bodybuilders and weightlifters was not attractive to most men and women, and even most athletes were reluctant to participate in serious strength training programs.

With the introduction of Nautilus equipment and the growth in the number of local fitness centers, strength training gained popularity and soon became the fastest growing activity in the field of exercise. This evolution was partly due to the ease of learning and using the Nautilus machines, and partly because the recommended training protocol (one set each of 10 to 12 exercises) was very time-efficient.

Like the running revolution that preceded it, many people who experienced the benefits of brief weight workouts assumed that more would be better. Influenced by increasingly popular physique magazines, large numbers of strength enthusiasts switched to free-weights and pursued more complex training protocols. These programs included split routines in which participants performed one-to-two hour training sessions, six days a week, working different muscle groups on different days.

While such training programs were typically effective for enhancing muscle and strength development, they presented two major problems for average men and women. First, the high volume of strength exercise resulted in a high rate of overuse injuries. Although heavily-muscled bodybuilders could tolerate the Herculean workouts, people with less musculoskeletal endowment experienced a variety of injuries to their muscles, tendons, fascia and joint structures.

The second concern involved the issue of time commitment. Even those who avoided or overcame physical injuries frequently found difficulty maintaining their training schedule. Unlike teenage trainees who can lift weights for a couple of hours after school, most adults are limited to before-work or after-work exercise sessions. Given the complex personal, professional, and social responsibilities of modern life, finding time for high-volume workouts became increasingly difficult for many individuals.

In response to these problematic issues, a number of strength professionals and exercise participants sought for an equally effective, but more time-efficient, training protocol that was high on results and low on injuries. Towards this end, Arthur Jones' high-intensity strength training techniques were revisited and researched to determine their suitability for satisfying these objectives.

When Arthur Jones developed and introduced Nautilus machines in the 1970s, he simultaneously set forth a series of basic training guidelines and fundamental exercise principles. These included relatively infrequent training sessions (two or three days per week), relatively few exercises (10 to 12 machines per workout), relatively brief training sessions (one set of eight to 12 repetitions per exercise), and relatively slow exercise speed (six seconds per repetition). After three decades of scrutiny and study, several professional certification associations presently support these basic strength-training principles, including the American College of Sports Medicine, the American Council on Exercise, the National Strength Professionals Association, and the YMCA of the USA.

At the same time, Jones presented more challenging exercise protocols for advanced trainees who desired even higher levels of muscle and strength development. These techniques included breakdown training, assisted training, pre-exhaustion training, and negative-only training. Because all of these exercise procedures were characterized by relatively high effort and short duration, they became known collectively as high-intensity strength training.

Generally speaking, a high-intensity training session will take you less than 30 minutes for completion. On the other hand, you will find it a physically demanding half-hour in terms of muscle effort. The basic concept for most high-intensity training techniques is to extend the exercise set in some way at the point of muscle fatigue to achieve an even greater strength-building stimulus. However, an equally productive procedure is to extend the exercise repetition by slowing down the movement speed. One technique, Super-Slow®, a method of training developed by Ken Hutchins, uses 10-second lifting movements and four-second lowering movements, thereby providing even more muscle tension on every repetition.

During the past several years, we have conducted many carefully controlled research studies on high-intensity strength training techniques. We have consistently found all of the exercise protocols to be both productive and efficient methods for enhancing muscle and strength development. High-intensity training has accelerated the rate of strength gain in beginners, and has enabled advanced exercisers to exceed previous strength plateaus.

You may wonder whether high-intensity training works with top athletes. In 1999, one of us had the privilege of speaking to the National Football League (NFL) strength coaches at their annual awards dinner. At that time, 10 of the 30 NFL teams trained *exclusively* with high-intensity strength exercise. This level of commitment is a pretty good indication that high-intensity training works at all levels of performance, as professional athletes from all sports will attest.

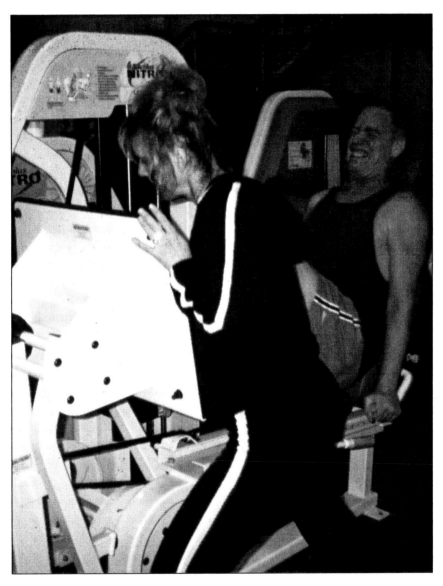

The basic concept underlying most high-intensity training techniques is to extend the exercise set in some way at the point of muscle fatigue to achieve an even greater strength-building stimulus.

As you read this book, you will learn how to properly perform all of the high-intensity training techniques, as well as how to combine procedures for even better results. You will also learn from the results of carefully controlled research studies what to expect from the various exercise protocols and the physiological reasons for their effectiveness.

Chapter One presents the physiological benefits related to extending the exercise set, particularly the recruitment and stimulus of additional muscle fibers. Chapter Two features *Breakdown Training* which is the basic means for extending the exercise set. Chapter Three then presents a detailed analysis of *Assisted Training*, which extends the exercise set more productively with the help of a partner. Chapter Four examines an even more comprehensive approach to extending the exercise set, called *Pre-Exhaustion Training*.

Chapter Five addresses the advantages associated with extending the exercise repetition, especially the greater sustained tension produced by the activated muscle fibers. The specifics of *Super Slow® Training* are presented in Chapter Six, with options for slow-positive or slow-negative exercise emphasis.

Chapter Seven discusses a *Combined Training Program* that includes one or two weeks of each high-intensity training technique for a more comprehensive exercise experience. Chapter Eight presents our most recent research on a *Combined Exercise Protocol* that has produced remarkable results with well-conditioned trainees. The book concludes with our recommendations for attaining the best possible results from high-intensity training. Chapter Nine addresses the importance of sufficient sleep, proper nutrition, and programmatic considerations such as training in the right repetition range for your muscle fiber make-up.

We sincerely hope that you will not only enjoy reading our research and recommendations on high-intensity training, but that you will experience excellent results from your personal exercise endeavors with these exciting procedures for maximum muscle conditioning.

W.L.W.

T.D.

1

Extending the Exercise Set

Whether you do single set or multiple set strength training, the predominant exercise pattern is to perform as many repetitions as possible to the point of muscle fatigue. A typical training set requires about eight to 12 repetitions with approximately 70 to 80 percent of maximum resistance. During the exercise set, muscle fibers are continuously recruited and fatigued until you have too few functioning muscle fibers to lift the resistance.

Let's examine the process a little more closely. Assume that you can perform one leg extension with 100 pounds, which represents your maximum resistance (1RM) for this exercise. You now place 75 pounds on the weightstack, which represents 75 percent of your 1RM. Using excellent exercise technique (i.e., slow-movement speed and full movement range), you complete 10 leg extensions before your quadriceps muscles reach fatigue and fail to lift the weightload. At this point, you do not have enough functioning muscle fiber to lift 75 percent of your maximum resistance. In other words, you are presently producing less than 75 percent of your maximum muscle strength, which means you have temporarily reduced your starting strength level by approximately 25 percent. Stated differently, you have fatigued about 25 percent of your quadriceps muscle fibers. The fatigued fibers have received a strength-building stimulus, and they will respond by becoming slightly larger and stronger, given sufficient rest and remodeling time.

Unfortunately, this standard training procedure does not provide a strength-building stimulus for the majority of muscle fibers which were not pushed to fatigue during the 10-repetition exercise set. While it is impossible to voluntarily fatigue all of the muscle fibers, there are training procedures that can increase the percentage of stimulated muscle fibers. These procedures, collectively called high-intensity strength training, use specific techniques to extend the exercise set. That is, upon reaching fatigue with the standard weightload, the resistance is reduced enough to complete a few more repetitions. By reaching a deeper level of fatigue, additional muscle fibers have experienced a strength-building stimulus, thereby enhancing muscle development.

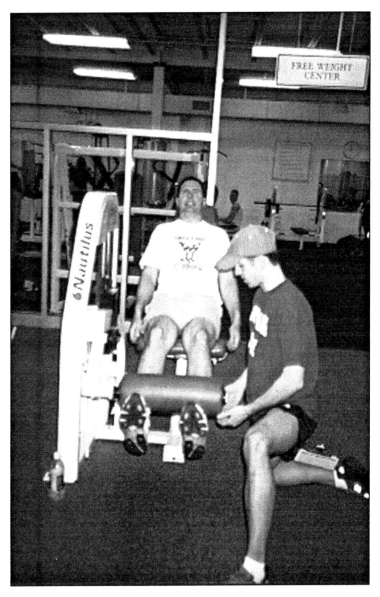

Reaching a deeper level of fatigue enables additional muscle fibers to experience a strength-building stimulus.

Slow-twitch and Fast-twitch Muscle Fibers

Your skeletal muscles are composed of two general types of fibers, known as slow-twitch and fast-twitch. The slow-twitch fibers have physiological characteristics that give them a high level of muscle endurance, meaning that they fatigue relatively slowly during use. Conversely, the fast-twitch fibers have physiological characteristics that give them a low level of muscle endurance, meaning that they fatigue quickly during use.

Although most of your major muscle groups have a fairly even mix of slow-twitch and fast-twitch muscle fibers, these are activated and fatigued in a very specific manner. When you are performing a standard exercise set, the more enduring slow-twitch muscle fibers are activated first and fatigue last. Just the opposite occurs with fast-twitch muscle fibers. The less enduring fast-twitch muscle fibers are activated last and fatigue first. Figure 1.1 provides a graphic representation of this process.

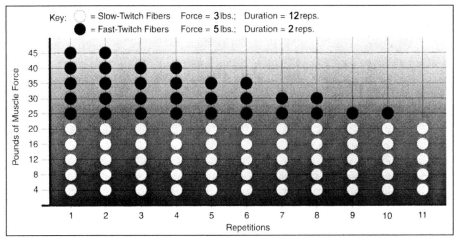

Figure 1.1 Hypothetical activation pattern of slow-twitch and fast-twitch muscle fibers during a set of 10 leg extensions with 25 pounds

As depicted in the illustration, assume that you have 10 muscle fibers in your quadriceps. Assume further that you have an even split of five slow-twitch and five fast-twitch muscle fibers. Let's say that each slow-twitch fiber can produce three pounds of force and can continue for 12 repetitions before fatiguing. Furthermore, let's assume that each fast-twitch fiber can produce five pounds of force, but can continue for only two repetitions before fatiguing.

You then place 20 pounds on the weightstack and begin a 10-repetition set of leg extensions. Your central nervous system (CNS) activates all five slow-twitch fibers, thereby generating 15 pounds of force which is insufficient to lift 20 pounds of resistance. Your CNS thereby activates one fast-twitch fiber, giving 20 pounds of force and enabling you to lift the weightload. After two repetitions, this particular fast-twitch fiber fatigues, and your CNS activates another fast-twitch fiber for the third and fourth repetitions. That fast-twitch fiber is then replaced by a new one for the fifth and sixth repetitions. Likewise, another fast-twitch fiber is recruited for the seventh and eighth repetitions. When this fast-twitch fiber fatigues, the last fast-twitch fiber is enrolled for the ninth and tenth repetitions. At this point, there are no more fresh fast-twitch fibers, and the slow-twitch fibers still produce only 15 pounds of force, so you cannot complete another repetition with the 20-pound weightload.

Although each fast-twitch muscle fiber was used for only two repetitions, they all worked to fatigue and experienced a strength-building stimulus. While each slow-twitch muscle fiber produced force for 10 consecutive repetitions, none reached the fatigue point necessary to attain a strength-building stimulus. Based on our hypothetical model, two more repetitions would be necessary to fatigue and stimulate some of the slow-twitch muscle fibers. By extending the exercise set for a few additional repetitions, this result could be achieved.

While this hypothetical example is somewhat simplified, it provides a reasonable portrayal of muscle-fiber activation patterns during a standard set of strength exercise. Studies on basic strength training consistently show that exercisers increase the size of their fast-twitch muscle fibers, but do not increase the size of their slow-twitch muscle fibers. On the other hand, muscle biopsies of top bodybuilders reveal an enlargement of both fast-twitch fibers and slow-twitch fibers. Apparently, the high-volume workouts of these body builders, characterized by lots of exercises, sets, repetitions, and hard training, impact both their fast-twitch and slow-twitch muscle fibers.

Unfortunately, most people do not have the time or physical ability to perform a typical bodybuilding training program. However, we have found that almost anyone can enhance strength and muscularity through relatively brief high-intensity training sessions. Although both men and women experience equivalent rates of strength gain, men typically add more muscle tissue due to their higher levels of testosterone.

The point to keep in mind is that extending the exercise set by a few repetitions adds only a little time to the workout duration, yet provides a productive means for stimulating both fast-twitch and slow-twitch muscle fibers for more strength building benefit.

You may wonder why it is not equally effective to simply use a lighter resistance and perform more repetitions per set. Such a procedure should certainly fatigue some of slow-twitch muscle fibers. However, lower weightloads reduce the exercise intensity for most of the repetitions and do not produce as much strength-building stimulus. By using a relatively heavy weightload to reach muscle fatigue within 60 seconds and then reducing the resistance to reach a deeper level of muscle fatigue within an additional 30 seconds, you complete a continuously challenging extended exercise set within the anaerobic energy system (approximately 90 seconds). Generally speaking, a weightload reduction of about 10 to 20 percent is recommended for achieving this desired result. Thus, extended-set training that incorporates two (or more) resistance levels is more effective than doing the same number of repetitions with a lighter weightload.

For most practical purposes, using an initial weightload that fatigues the target muscles within eight to 10 repetitions is recommended. At a repetition speed of six seconds for each repetitive (two seconds lifting and four seconds lowering), the first level of muscle fatigue should occur within 48 to 60 seconds. At this point, the resistance should be reduced enough to permit two to five additional repetitions. In this manner, the extended set should be completed within 60 to 90 seconds, and provide greater strength building stimulus by fatiguing more muscle fibers with relatively heavy resistance.

Of course, it is possible to reduce the resistance more than once and extend the exercise set beyond the anaerobic energy system. Doing this increases both the exercise time and the muscle discomfort, which may result in overtraining, reduced strength gains, and burnout. Too much microtrauma to the muscle tissue can be counterproductive, by employing more recovery energy for repair purposes than for building processes.

Extended-Set Training Techniques

Three basic procedures exist for effectively extending the exercise set, namely, breakdown training, assisted training, and pre-exhaustion training. All three high-intensity training techniques require you to perform a few post-fatigue repetitions, but these are done in different ways. In breakdown training, you simply lower the weightload upon reaching muscle fatigue. In assisted training, you utilize a partner to help lift the resistance when it exceeds your muscle's reduced strength levels. In pre-exhaustion training, you combine two successive exercises for the target muscle group. Each extended-set training technique will be addressed separately and specifically in the three following chapters.

Whichever technique you use, your training outcomes will be better if you pay strict attention to your exercise form. This guideline includes proper posture throughout each training set, full movement range on every repetition, and slow movement speed on every repetition. Incorporating these form factors enhances muscle isolation and intensity, thereby increasing the strength-building stimulus.

Make Every Repetition Count

Keep in mind that because high-intensity strength workouts typically require only one set of each exercise, it is essential to make every repetition count. With respect to the target muscles, good form enhances good effort. Both are key components for best results.

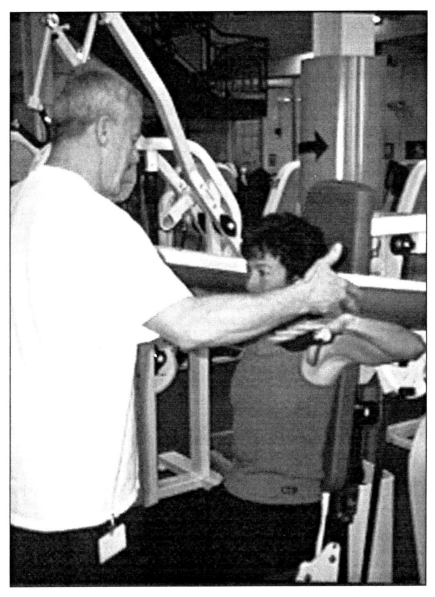

For most practical purposes, using an initial weightload that fatigues the target muscles within eight to ten repetitions is recommended.

2

Breakdown Training

The simplest means for extending the exercise set is known as breakdown training. As the name implies, you break down the level of resistance as your muscle strength breaks down in order to continue the exercise set. That is, when the muscles can no longer lift the initial weightload, it is reduced sufficiently enough to enable a few post-fatigue repetitions. As was discussed in the previous chapter, this procedure produces two levels of muscle fatigue and stimulates some of the more enduring slow-twitch muscle fibers.

How It Works

The first step in breakdown training is to select a weightload that can be lifted for about 8 to 10 good repetitions. Each repetition should be performed through a full-movement range at a slow-movement speed. Two seconds for each lifting movement (concentric muscle action) and four seconds for each lowering movement (eccentric muscle action), which totals six seconds per repetition and 48 to 60 seconds per set are recommended. The initial set typically uses about 75 percent of maximum resistance and is terminated at the point of muscle fatigue when the starting strength has been reduced by about 25 percent. At this point, the majority of fatigued and stimulated muscle fibers are the low endurance fast-twitch fibers.

The second step in breakdown training is to immediately reduce the resistance by 10 to 20 percent when the initial weightload can no longer be lifted. Without resting, complete as many repetitions as possible with the lighter weightload to reach a second level of muscle fatigue. This extended segment of the set usually requires two to five additional repetitions, and stimulates some of the high-endurance, slow-twitch muscle fibers.

Note that the time requirement for the 10 to 15 total repetitions is between 60 and 90 seconds, which is within the anaerobic energy system. The optimum strength-building stimulus is attained when the high-intensity training set is completed in the end range of the anaerobic energy system, which occurs at roughly 60 to 90 seconds.

When using machines, you can quickly reduce the resistance by pulling the pin and reinserting it in the weightstack at the desired level. When using free-weights, simply pick-up a lighter set of dumbbells or slide the appropriate plates (e.g., 5 lbs, 10 lbs, etc.) off both ends of the barbell.

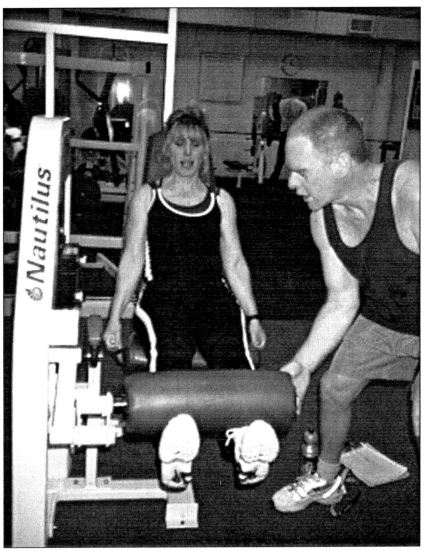

The simplest means for extending an exercise set is known as breakdown training.

Research on Breakdown Training

We generally conduct our high-intensity research studies with both beginning and advanced participants. Beginning participants present an equitable baseline measure, or even playing field, because they do not have prior strength training experience or personal biases towards certain exercise techniques. We therefore compare two groups of beginning subjects in our research—one group that does the standard strength training program with a matched group that performs the desired high-intensity strength-training program.

Because advanced trainees have widely varying exercise experiences and abilities, it is extremely difficult to find matched groups for comparative purposes. For this reason, we use advanced trainees as their own controls. That is, they are required to perform standard strength training for some muscle groups, and high-intensity strength training for unrelated muscle groups. In reality, well-designed self-comparisons provide the most valid information about the effects of different strength training techniques in advanced participants.

Beginning Subjects

In one particular study that we conducted, 45 previously untrained men and women were randomly assigned to one of two exercise groups. During the first month, both groups did standard strength training on the following Nautilus machines: leg extension, leg curl, leg press, chest cross, pullover, lateral raise, biceps curl, triceps extension, low back, abdominal and neck. That is, all of the subjects performed each exercise for one set of eight to 12 repetitions, using approximately 75 percent of their maximum resistance. Whenever they completed 12 good repetitions (i.e., full-movement range and slow-movement speed), the weightload was increased by about five percent (2.5 to 5.0 pounds) for the next workout.

During the second month of the study, Group #1 continued to train with the standard exercise procedures. However, Group #2 performed breakdown training on the leg curl and abdominal machines. When they reached the point of muscle fatigue on these exercises, the weightload was reduced by 10 pounds, and they performed as many additional repetitions as possible with the lighter resistance. Because almost all of the participants used between 50 and 100 pounds in the leg curl and abdominal exercises, the 10-pound weightstack reduction represented about 10 to 20 percent less resistance for the post-fatigue repetitions. On average, the subjects completed three additional repetitions with the reduced resistance.

At the conclusion of the three-days-per-week exercise program, the subjects who completed two months of standard training increased their 10-repetition maximum

(10RM) weightloads on the leg curl and abdominal machines by an average of 18 pounds. By comparison, the subjects who performed one month of standard training and one month of breakdown training increased their 10RM weightloads on the leg curl and abdominal machines by an average of 25 pounds.

As presented graphically in Figure 2.1, the breakdown training group experienced 40-percent greater strength gains than the standard training group. Because all other aspects of the two exercise programs were identical, it would appear that breakdown training is more effective than standard training for developing muscle strength in beginning participants.

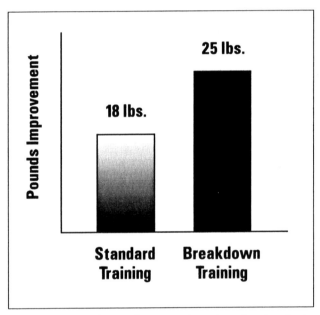

Figure 2.1 Eight-week strength gains for beginning subjects using standard and breakdown training (N=45)

Advanced Subjects

In a smaller-scale study with advanced exercisers, seven men and women performed breakdown training on Nautilus machines twice-a-week for a period of six weeks under close supervision of a personal trainer. Their strength increases in the breakdown training exercises (leg extension, biceps curl, and weight-assisted chin-up) were compared to their strength increases in the standard training exercises (low back and abdominal).

As shown in Figure 2.2, these advanced subjects increased their average 10 RM weightloads by 15 pounds in their breakdown-training exercises and by 12 pounds in their standard-training exercises. Although the relatively small number of research subjects ruled out statistical analyses, breakdown training produced 25 percent greater strength gains in these seasoned participants. It would therefore appear that breakdown training is an effective strength building technique for advanced, as well as beginning, exercisers.

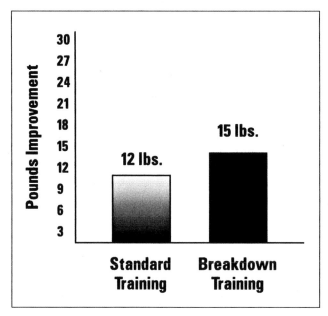

Figure 2.2 Six-week strength gains for advanced subjects using standard and breakdown training (N=7)

In a more recent study, 11 moderately-conditioned men and women did six weeks of twice-a-week breakdown training. They performed eight repetitions to fatigue, followed immediately by four post-fatigue repetitions with 10 to 20 percent less resistance using the following twelve exercises:

- leg curl
- leg press
- chest cross
- chest press
- pullover
- pulldown
- lateral raise
- shoulder press
- biceps curl
- triceps extension
- abdominal curl
- low-back extension

As presented in Table 2.1, the participants significantly surpassed their previous best performances in both weightstack exercises (which they did each workout) and bodyweight exercises (which they did not do during the study period). These results provide further evidence that breakdown training is a productive procedure for overcoming strength plateaus.

Table 2.1 Six-week performance improvements for moderately conditioned subjects using breakdown training (N = 11)

Lateral Raise Weightload	Chin-Ups	Bar-Dips
+ 13.9 lbs	+ 1.5 reps	+ 2.5 reps
(51.2 lbs - 65.1 lbs)	(2.2 reps - 3.7 reps)	(5.5 reps - 8.0 reps)

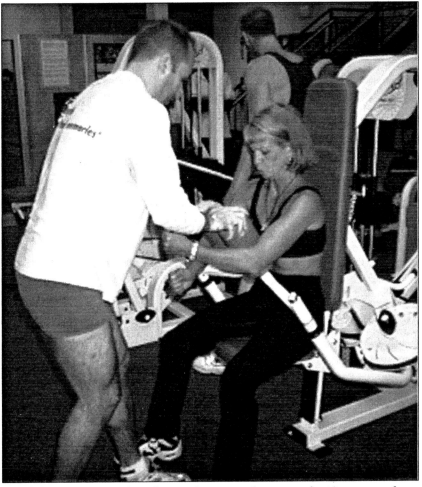

Breakdown training has been shown to be a productive procedure for overcoming strength plateaus.

Concluding Comments

Breakdown training is the most basic procedure for extending the exercise set. Although it can be performed on most types of equipment, breakdown training is most easily adapted to weightstack machines. By simply removing and reinserting the pin, the resistance can be quickly reduced by 10 to 20 percent. This relatively rapid transition prevents the fatigued fast-twitch muscle fibers from recovering, and forces some of the more enduring slow-twitch muscle fibers to reach fatigue. In this manner, a well-executed set of breakdown training results in more fatigued muscle fibers (fast-twitch and slow-twitch) and a greater strength-building stimulus.

Although it is possible to do additional breakdowns, a single reduction in the initial exercise resistance is recommended for most practical purposes. A breakdown set that permits eight to 10 repetitions to the first level of fatigue (48 to 60 seconds) and two to five repetitions to the second level of fatigue (12 to 30 seconds) is highly effective for increasing muscle strength. Doing additional breakdown repetitions at this point may extend the exercise set beyond the timeframe in which the anaerobic energy system is involved (90 seconds) and cause considerable physical discomfort, which can adversely affect the training process and product. Breakdown training can be applied to all exercises and all muscle groups. However, because it is a more demanding training procedure, you will need more recovery time between exercise sessions for your muscles to rebuild and achieve greater strength capacity. Generally speaking, two breakdown workouts per week are sufficient for a high rate of strength gain and muscle development. A Monday and Friday sequence is recommended, with quality rest and good nutrition throughout the training period.

After six weeks of breakdown training, you should see significant improvements in your level of muscle strength. However, to reduce the risk of burnout, you should return to standard training for an equivalent length of time. This step permits a reasonable adjustment period to the higher-strength levels and helps reduce your risk of being affected by an overtraining syndrome. After six weeks of standard training, a return to breakdown training should be well-received physiologically and psychologically, with further gains in muscle strength occurring.

Table 2.2 presents a sample program of breakdown training for intermediate level participants with realistic examples of the exercises, muscle groups, initial weightloads for pre-fatigue repetitions and reduced weightloads for post-fatigue repetitions. In this hypothetical protocol, the initial weightloads are reduced by 15 percent for the post-fatigue repetitions.

Table 2.2 An example of a breakdown training program for intermediate level participants, with sample exercises, muscle groups, and suggested weightloads for both the pre-fatigue and post-fatigue repetitions

Sample Exercises	Muscle Groups	Initial Weightload For Pre-Fatigue Reps*	Reduced Weightload for Post-Fatigue Reps**
Hip Adduction	Hip Adductors	140 lbs x 8-10 reps	120 lbs x 3-5 reps
Hip Abduction	Hip Abductors	100 lbs x 8-10 reps	85 lbs x 3-5 reps
Leg Press	Quadriceps Hamstrings Gluteals	200 lbs x 8-10 reps	170 lbs x 3-5 reps
Chest Press	Pectorals Major	120 lbs x 8-10 reps	100 lbs x 3-5 reps
Seated Row	Latissimus Dorsi	140 lbs x 8-10 reps	120 lbs x 3-5 reps
Shoulder Press	Deltoids	100 lbs x 8-10 reps	85 lbs x 3-5 reps
Low Back	Erector Spinae	100 lbs x 8-10 reps	85 lbs x 3-5 reps
Abdominal	Rectus Abdominis	80 lbs x 8-10 reps	70 lbs x 3-5 reps
Rotary Torso	Internal Obliques External Obliques	60 lbs x 8-10 reps	50 lbs x 3-5 reps

*Note: When 11 repetitions can be properly performed, the exercise resistance is increased by five percent or less.

**Note: When six repetitions can be properly performed, the exercise resistance is increased by five percent or less.

3

Assisted Training

Another means for extending the exercise set is called assisted training. As the name infers, this high-intensity technique incorporates an assistant to help you complete a few post-fatigue repetitions. That is, when your muscles can no longer lift the exercise weightload, a partner provides as much manual assistance as necessary for two to five additional repetitions. As was discussed in Chapter One, this procedure produces multiple levels of muscle fatigue and stimulates strength development in some of the more enduring, slow-twitch muscle fibers.

Beyond Breakdown Training

Although assisted training is similar to breakdown training in theory, two important differences exist between these two extended-set exercise techniques. The first difference is that assisted training requires a knowledgeable and cooperative partner/trainer to give appropriate assistance when you reach muscle fatigue.

The second difference is that a well-executed set of assisted training produces eccentric-muscle fatigue as well as concentric-muscle fatigue. As you may be aware, your eccentric-muscle actions are about 40 percent stronger than your concentric muscle actions. For this reason, you can lower approximately 40 percent more weight under control than you can lift. In other words, if you can lift 100 pounds in the leg extension exercise you can actually lower 140 pounds at the same controlled movement speed.

In breakdown training, the resistance is reduced by 10 to 20 percent when your muscles can no longer lift the initial weightload. While a lighter weightload is necessary for post-fatigue lifting movements, the initial resistance can still be lowered under control for a few more repetitions. This feature is the primary advantage of assisted training. The assistant gives only as much help as necessary on the post-fatigue lifting movements, and no help on the post-fatigue lowering movements.

After a few assisted repetitions, muscle strength is reduced below the level required for controlled lowering movements, and a degree of eccentric muscle fatigue is experienced. This factor makes assisted training a more challenging means for extending the exercise set, and a procedure that has produced excellent results in our research studies.

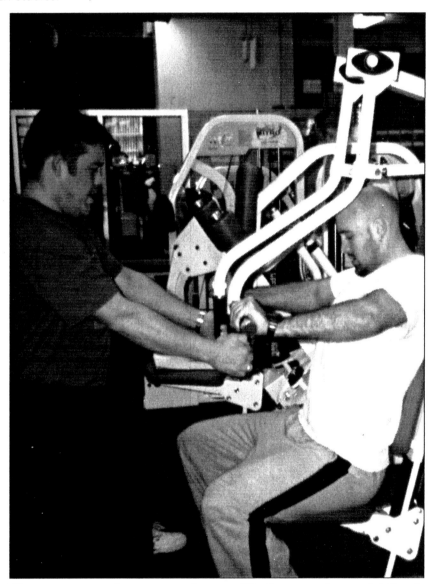

When your muscles can no longer lift the exercise weightload, assisted training involves having a partner provide as much manual assistance as necessary for you to perform two to five additional repetitions.

How It Works

The first step in assisted training is to select a weightload that can be lifted for about eight to 10 good repetitions. Each repetition should be performed through a full-movement range at a slow-movement speed. You should take two seconds for each lifting movement (concentric muscle action) and four seconds for each lowering movement (eccentric muscle action), (a total of six seconds per repetition and 48 to 60 seconds per set). The initial set typically uses about 75 percent of maximum resistance and is terminated at the point of muscle fatigue, when your starting strength has been reduced by about 25 percent. At this point, the majority of stimulated muscle fibers are the quick-to-fatigue, fast-twitch fibers.

The next step in assisted training is to receive manual assistance from a partner when the initial weightload can no longer be lifted. Give as much force as you can, while your partner makes up the difference to complete each post-fatigue lifting movement. Give as much force as necessary to control each post-fatigue, lowering movement. Two to five assisted repetitions are usually sufficient to reach deeper levels of muscle fatigue and stimulate strength development in some of the more enduring slow-twitch muscle fibers.

Note that the time requirement for the 10 to 15 total repetitions is between 60 and 90 seconds, which is within the anaerobic energy system. Keep in mind that your optimum strength-building stimulus is attained when you complete the high-intensity training set in the end range of your anaerobic energy system (i.e., 60 to 90 seconds).

Research on Assisted Training

As was stated in Chapter 2, we typically conduct our high-intensity research studies with both beginning and advanced participants. Our studies with beginners incorporate two exercise groups, one that performs the standard strength-training program and one that performs the desired high-intensity strength training program.

Our studies with advanced trainees use the same subjects to compare the effects of different exercise protocols. In these investigative undertakings, the participants perform standard strength training for some muscle groups, and high-intensity strength training for unrelated muscle groups.

Beginning Subjects

In this study, which was similar to the study on breakdown training, 42 previously sedentary men and women were randomly assigned to one of two exercise groups.

During the first month of the study, both groups did standard strength training on the following Nautilus machines: leg extension, leg curl, leg press, chest cross, pullover, lateral raise, biceps curl, triceps extension, low back, abdominal, and neck. The protocol for this study required all of the subjects to perform each exercise for one set of eight to 12 repetitions using approximately 75 percent of their maximum resistance. Whenever they completed 12 repetitions in good form (full movement range and slow movement speed), the weightload was increased by about five percent (2.5 to 5.0 pounds) for the next workout.

During the second month, Group #1 continued to train with standard exercise procedures. However, Group #2 performed assisted training on the leg curl and abdominal machines. When they reached the point of muscle fatigue on these exercises, they received manual assistance from an instructor. The instructor helped with the lifting phase, but not the lowering phase, of three post-fatigue repetitions.

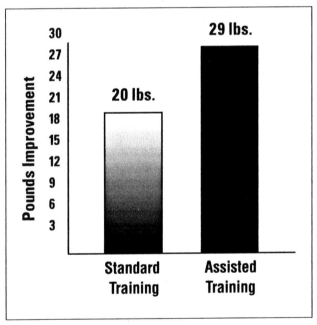

Figure 3.1 Eight-week strength gains for beginning subjects using standard and assisted training (N=42)

At the conclusion of the three-days-per-week exercise program, the subjects who completed two months of standard training increased their 10-repetition maximum (10 RM) weightloads on the leg curl and abdominal machines by an average of 20 pounds. By comparison, the subjects who performed one month of standard training and one month of assisted training increased their 10 RM weightloads on the leg curl and abdominal machines by an average of 29 pounds.

As shown graphically in Figure 3.1, the assisted training group experienced 45-percent greater strength gains than the standard training group. Because all other aspects of the two exercise programs were identical, it would appear that assisted training is more effective than standard training for developing muscle strength in beginning participants.

Advanced Subjects

In a smaller scale study with advanced exercisers, seven men and women performed assisted training on Nautilus machines twice-a-week for a period of six weeks with help from a personal trainer. The strength increases experienced by these subjects in the assisted training exercises (leg curl, triceps extension, and weight assisted bar-dip) were then compared to their strength increases in the standard training exercises (low back and abdominal).

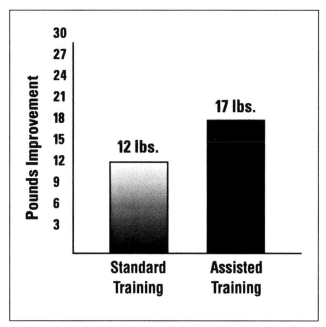

Figure 3.2 Six week strength gains for advanced subjects using standard and assisted training (N=7)

As presented in Figure 3.2, these advanced subjects increased their 10 RM weightload by 17 pounds in their assisted training exercises and by 12 pounds in their standard training exercises. Although the relatively small number of research subjects ruled out statistical analyses, assisted training produced 40-percent greater strength gains than standard training in these experienced exercisers. It would therefore appear that assisted training is an effective strength building technique for advanced, as well as beginning, exercisers.

In another study that involved previously trained participants, 15 men and women did five weeks of twice-a-week assisted training. The subjects performed eight repetitions to fatigue, followed immediately by four post-fatigue assisted repetitions, using the following exercises:

- leg curl
- leg press
- chest cross
- chest press
- pullover
- pulldown

- lateral raise
- shoulder press
- biceps curl
- triceps extension
- abdominal curl
- low back extension

As presented in Table 3.1, the subjects made significant performance improvements in both weightstack exercises (which they did each workout) and bodyweight exercises (which they did not do during the study period). These results further support assisted training as a productive procedure for overcoming strength plateaus.

Table 3.1 Five-week performance improvements for advanced subjects using assisted training (N = 15)

Lateral Raise Weightload	Chin-Ups	Bar-Dips
+ 10.6 lbs	+ 1.4 reps	+ 4.5 reps
(66.2 lbs - 76.8 lbs)	(4.7 reps - 6.1 reps)	(9.6 reps - 14.1 reps)

Concluding Comments

Assisted training is a somewhat more complex and challenging means for extending the exercise set. A competent and cooperative partner/trainer provides assistance on the post-fatigue lifting movements but not on the post-fatigue lowering movements. A well-executed set of assisted training therefore produces a high level of concentric muscle fatigue, as well as a degree of eccentric muscle fatigue when the exerciser has difficulty controlling the lowering movement.

Assisted training can be performed with essentially all forms of resistance exercise, including machines, free-weights, and even bodyweight. It is perhaps easiest to assist on machines, because the movement pattern is typically fixed and does not require manual guidance or control.

Although it is possible to give more than five assisted lifts, performing more than five is usually unnecessary. By the fifth post-fatigue repetition, the exerciser generally has difficulty controlling the lowering movement, which indicates a high level of eccentric muscle fatigue. More post-fatigue repetitions can also cause considerable discomfort, which may be counter-productive from a psychological perspective. Also, doing additional repetitions at this point may extend the exercise set beyond the time limits imposed by your anaerobic energy system (i.e., 90 seconds).

Like breakdown training, assisted training can be applied to all exercises and all muscle groups. However, the greater physical demands of this high-intensity training procedure requires more recovery time between exercise sessions for your muscles to rebuild and achieve higher strength levels. Typically, two assisted workouts per week are sufficient for significant strength gains. We have achieved excellent results with a Monday-and-Friday sequence, with quality rest and good nutrition throughout the training period.

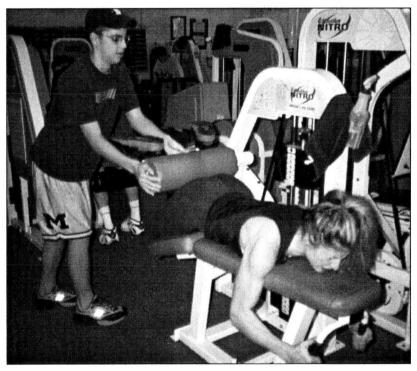

Assisted training can be performed with essentially all forms of resistance exercise, including machines, free weights, and even body weight.

After six weeks of assisted training, you should observe significant improvements in muscle development. At this point, you should return to standard training for an equivalent length of time to reduce the risk of overtraining. This schedule permits a reasonable adjustment period to the higher strength levels and reduces your risk of burnout. After six weeks of standard training, you should be fresh physiologically and psychologically for another productive six-week program of assisted training.

Because it is impossible to determine how many pounds of assistance the partner provides during the post-fatigue repetitions, a sample assisted training workout cannot accurately be detailed. Suffice to say that the initial weightload should be heavy enough to fatigue the target muscles within eight to 10 repetitions, followed by as little assistance as necessary for performing up to five additional repetitions. At the point where you can no longer control a four-second lowering movement (eccentric muscle action), the set should be terminated, even if this occurs on the second or third post-fatigue repetition.

4

Pre-Exhaustion Training

A third and somewhat more interesting method for extending the exercise set is known as pre-exhaustion training. Actually, pre-exhaustion training involves two successive sets of different exercises for the same target muscle group, but without resting between exercises. The idea is to work the target muscle to fatigue with one exercise, then to push it to a deeper level of strength-building stimulus with another exercise.

How It Works

L ext   rotary-curved-single
press/pull leg press,   linear-straight - more than one mm

While pre-exhaustion training may be approached in numerous ways using various pairs of exercises, it seems to work best when addressed in the following manner. The first step is to select a rotary (curved movement) exercise that isolates the target muscle. For example, the leg extension is a rotary exercise that essentially isolates the quadriceps muscles.

The second step is to use a weightload that fatigues the target muscle within eight to 10 good repetitions (i.e., slow-movement speed through full-movement range). Assume that you can perform 10 leg extensions with 100 pounds to the point of muscle fatigue (inability to complete another lifting movement). At this point, your quadriceps muscles have experienced about 60 seconds of high-effort, anaerobic exercise that has fatigued and stimulated many of the fast-twitch muscle fibers.

The third step is to perform another exercise that works the target (quadriceps) muscle. To prevent the fatigued fast-twitch fibers from recovering, the second exercise should be performed with as little delay as possible. To enable a reasonably heavy level of resistance to be used, the second exercise should be linear (straight movement). Linear exercises include pressing and pulling actions that involve two or more major muscle groups. For example, the leg press is a linear exercise that incorporates both the quadriceps and hamstrings muscles.

The fourth (and final) step is to use a weightload that permits only four to five good repetitions. Because the quadriceps muscles are already fatigued, the leg press resistance must be reduced accordingly. However, the fresh hamstring muscles assist the pre-fatigued quadriceps muscles, thereby enabling you to perform a few high-effort leg presses that fatigue even more of the quadriceps' slow-twitch muscle fibers. This procedure produces a significant strength-building stimulus that enhances quadriceps development beyond standard training.

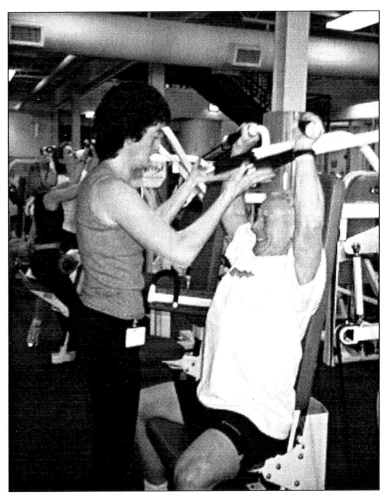

Pre-exhaustion training involves performing two successive sets of different exercises for the same target muscle group, but without resting between exercises.

Assume, for example, that you can now perform only five leg presses with 200 pounds, which requires about 30 seconds. You have now completed about 90 seconds of quadriceps training between the two successive exercises (10 leg extensions in 60 seconds, followed by five leg presses in 30 seconds). The result is a deep level of quadriceps fatigue within the time parameters of your anaerobic energy system (90 seconds) that should activate a growth response in both your fast-twitch muscle fibers (primarily stimulated in the first exercise) and your slow-twitch muscle fibers (primarily stimulated in the second exercise).

As you can see, following a rotary (single muscle) exercise with a linear (multiple muscle) exercise brings in fresh assisting muscles to push the target muscles to a higher level of fatigue and provide a greater strength-building stimulus. In addition, pre-exhaustion training involves two separate exercises with specific movement patterns that incorporate different muscle fibers within the target muscles. Pre-exhaustion training also offers a psychological benefit, because the post-fatigue repetitions are performed with a different exercise than was employed for the pre-fatigue repetitions. In other words, instead of completing more repetitions of the same exercise with a reduced resistance as in breakdown and assisted training, you experience a welcome change in the movement pattern. Keep in mind that the less time taken between the two exercises, the greater the training effect on the target muscle group.

Research on Pre-Exhaustion Training

Our research on pre-exhaustion training has been limited to intermediate and advanced subjects. In the first study we conducted on pre-exhaustion training, we simply compared pre-exhaustion training with multiple-set training. While pre-exhaustion procedures require two sets (one set each of two different exercises) for the target muscles, a major difference exists between this approach to training and multi-set training. Unlike standard multiple-set training, pre-exhaustion training allows very little recovery time between the successive sets of exercise. This factor provides at least two advantages. First, the fatigued fast-twitch muscle fibers are unable to participate in the second exercise, thereby forcing the more enduring slow-twitch muscle fibers to attain a training stimulus. Second, because the two-minute rest generally taken between repeat exercise sets is eliminated, the pre-exhaustion training session is much more time-efficient.

Consider, for example, the time difference involved in performing a set of 10 leg extensions followed by a set of five leg presses compared to performing two standard sets of 10 leg extensions each. Two pre-exhaustion exercises for the quadriceps muscles require about 100 seconds (60 seconds for 10 leg extensions, 10 seconds transfer time between machines, and 30 seconds for five leg presses). Two standard exercise sets for the quadriceps muscles typically require about 210 seconds (60 seconds for 10 leg extensions, 90 seconds recovery time between sets, and 60 seconds for 10 leg extensions), which is more than twice the training time compared to pre-exhaustion exercise.

Intermediate Subjects

The subjects in this study were 14 men and women who trained on 12 Nautilus machines under close instructor supervision, two times per week for a period of six weeks. All of the participants performed pre-exhaustion training for the pectorals major muscles (10 chest crosses, followed immediately by five chest presses) and for the triceps muscles (10 triceps extensions, followed immediately by five bar-dips). They all performed multiple-set training for the latissimus dorsi muscles (two sets of 10 super pullovers, with 90 seconds rest between sets) and for the biceps muscles (two sets of 10 biceps curls, with 90 seconds rest between sets). All of the other Nautilus exercises were performed in the standard manner (one set of eight to 12 repetitions).

As illustrated in Figure 4.1, the pre-exhaustion training produced an average 8.5-pound strength gain in the pectoralis major and triceps exercises. Interestingly, the multiple-set training produced an average 8.5-pound strength gain in the latissimus dorsi and biceps exercises. In other words, the two training techniques elicited essentially the same rate of strength development in these opposing muscle groups (pectoralis major vs latissimus dorsi and triceps vs biceps). However, the pre-exhaustion training was completed in less than half the time required for the multiple-set training (100 seconds vs 210 seconds per target muscle group). Although this study did not prove one training technique to be more effective than the other, it clearly demonstrated that pre-exhaustion training is more time-efficient than multiple-set training. For time-pressured people, training efficiency is an essential consideration in successful workout design.

Advanced Subjects

In another study, we examined the effects of pre-exhaustion training on both muscle strength and body composition in more advanced exercisers. The 16 adult participants performed two full-body pre-exhaustion workouts per week for a period of six weeks. Each training session was carefully supervised by an instructor and included the following sixteen exercises: leg extension; leg curl; leg press; chest cross; bench press; pullover; pulldown; lateral raise; overhead press; biceps curl; chin-up; triceps extension; bar dip; low back; abdominal; and rotary torso. Due to the brief recovery periods between exercises, the total training time for each pre-exhaustion workout was less than 30 minutes.

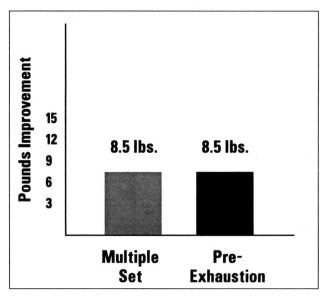

Figure 4.1 Six-week strength gains for intermediate subjects, using multiple-set and pre-exhaustion training (N=14). Due to 90-second rest period between successive sets, the multiple-set exercise bouts required about 210 seconds, whereas the pre-exhaustion exercise bouts required about 100 seconds.

After 12 pre-exhaustion training sessions that addressed the major muscle groups, the subjects experienced a 15-pound average increase in their exercise weightloads. In addition, the pre-exhaustion workouts produced an average lean (muscle) weight gain of 2.2 pounds and an average fat weight loss of 2.1 pounds. Although their bodyweight remained the same, the trainees made a four-pound change in their body composition. These impressive physical improvements can be almost exclusively attributed to the pre-exhaustion training program, since no other aspects of the subjects' lifestyle (e.g., diet, endurance exercise, etc.) were altered during the study. Figure 4.2 presents the results of this study graphically.

Concluding Comments

Pre-exhaustion training is a very interesting means for extending the exercise set that can be performed effectively on most types of equipment. However, it appears to work best when the exercises are paired in the following manner: a rotary exercise that isolates the target muscle, followed immediately by a linear exercise that brings in a fresh assisting muscle to further fatigue the target muscle. A quick transition between successive exercises prevents the pre-fatigued, fast-twitch muscle fibers from recovering and forces some of the more enduring slow-twitch muscle fibers to reach

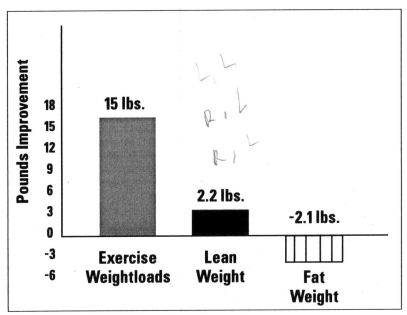

Figure 4.2 Six-week strength changes in exercise weightloads, lean weight, and fat weight for advanced subjects using pre-exhaustion training (N=16)

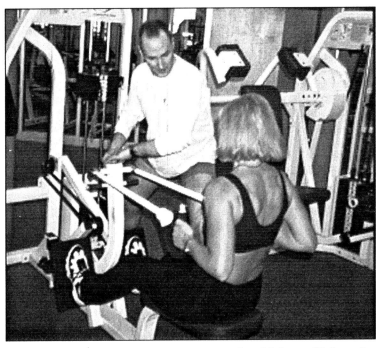

Six weeks of pre-exhaustion training should be sufficient for achieving significant improvements in both muscle strength and body composition.

Table 4.1 An example of a pre-exhaustion training program for advanced level participants with sample exercises, muscle groups, and suggested weightloads for both the first and second exercises.

Sample Exercises	Muscle Groups	Suggested Weightloads for First Exercise*	Suggested Weightloads for Second Exercise**
Leg Extension	Quadriceps	150 lbs x 10 reps	
Leg Press	Quadriceps Hamstrings		300 lbs x 5 reps
Leg Curl	Hamstrings	125 lbs x 10 reps	
Hip Extension	Hamstrings Gluteals		150 lbs x 5 reps
Chest Cross	Pectoralis Major	125 lbs x 10 reps	
Chest Press	Pectoralis Major Triceps		175 lbs x 5 reps
Pullover	Latissimus Dorsi	150 lbs x 10 reps	
Pulldown	Latissimus Dorsi Biceps		200 lbs x 5 reps
Lateral Raise	Deltoids	100 lbs x 10 reps	
Shoulder Pres	Deltoids Triceps		150 lbs x 5 reps
Biceps Curl	Biceps	75 lbs x 10 reps	
Wt. Assist Chin-Up	Biceps Latissimus Dorsi		50 lbs x 5 reps
Triceps Extension	Triceps	75 lbs x 10 reps	
Wt. Assist. Bar Dip	Triceps Pectoralis Major		50 lbs x 5 reps
Low Back	Erector Spinae	150 lbs x 10 reps	(one exercise only)
Abdominal	Rectus Abdominis	125 lbs x 10 reps	(one exercise only)

*Note: When 11 repetitions can be properly performed, the exercise resistance is increased by five percent or less.

**Note: When six repetitions can be properly performed, the exercise resistance is increased by five percent or less.

fatigue. A properly performed sequence of pre-exhaustion exercises results in more fatigued muscle fibers (both fast-twitch and slow-twitch) for a greater strength-building stimulus.

Under some circumstances, well-conditioned trainees may perform three successive exercises for the target muscle group. However, this approach may lead to overtraining and is not recommended for most practical purposes. A pre-exhaustion combination that uses a rotary exercise to fatigue the target muscle in eight to 10 repetitions (48 to 60 seconds), followed by a linear exercise that further fatigues the target muscle in four to five repetitions (24 to 30 seconds) is highly effective for increasing muscle strength and size. Adding a third exercise at this point may work the muscle beyond the anaerobic energy system (90 seconds) and create considerable physical discomfort, both of which can reduce training effectiveness.

While you may apply pre-exhaustion training to most of your major muscle groups, you should make a few exceptions in this regard. For example, for safety sake, you should not perform pre-exhaustion procedures on more vulnerable body parts, such as the low back and neck muscles. Because pre-exhaustion training is a more complex and challenging exercise technique, your muscles will require longer recovery periods to rebuild and attain higher strength levels between workouts.

Six weeks of pre-exhaustion training should be sufficient for achieving significant improvements in both muscle strength and body composition. Although longer training periods may produce even better results, six weeks of pre-exhaustion training, followed by six weeks of standard training to reduce the risk of burnout, are recommended. After six weeks of standard training, you may return to the same pre-exhaustion procedures or design different pairs of rotary and linear exercises to stimulate additional muscle development.

Table 4.1 offers a sample program of pre-exhaustion training for advanced level participants with realistic examples of the exercises, muscle groups, weightloads for the first (rotary) exercise, and weightloads for the second (linear) exercise. In reality, the resistance level used in the first exercise should permit about eight to 10 repetitions, while the resistance level employed in the second exercise should permit about four to five repetitions.

5

Extending the Exercise Repetition—Slow Training

If you are like most people, you began strength training with a basic program of 10 to 15 exercises which you performed for one set of eight to 12 repetitions each. This training protocol probably produced progressive strength gains for several weeks or months. However, you eventually experienced a strength plateau and failed to see further improvement. At this point, you may have been advised to do more exercises for each muscle group or to do more sets of each exercise.

While these are useful recommendations, they may not be practical for all exercise participants, particularly those who have time restrictions. Exercisers who want to progress further or faster in a time-efficient manner should consider high-intensity training techniques. These training procedures produce higher levels of muscle conditioning within essentially the same time frame as a basic strength training program.

The primary purpose of high-intensity strength training is to make each exercise set more challenging to your target muscles. One simple but highly effective means for accomplishing this objective is to extend the exercise repetition by using a slower-movement speed.

As illustrated in Figure 5.1, slower movement speeds produce more muscle tension (represented by the total area within each strength-curve tracing) and greater muscle force (represented by the height of each strength-curve tracing). For example, the maximum quadriceps force (Q tracing) produced by this individual in a knee extension at the relatively slow speed of 60 degrees per second is 174 foot-pounds. However, the maximum quadriceps force produced by the same individual in a knee extension at the relatively fast speed of 120 degrees per second is only 132 foot-pounds.

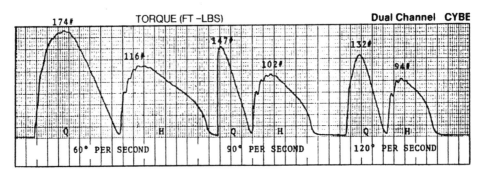

Figure 5.1 Comparison of muscle tension (area under each strength curve tracing) and muscle force (height of each strength curve tracing) at three movement speeds from Cybex II isokinetic strength assessment

Q = quadriceps and H = hamstrings.

Because procedures that produce more muscle tension and greater muscle force enhance strength development, slower exercise speeds are preferable to faster exercise speeds. Although faster movement speeds permit the use of heavier weightloads, this factor is largely the result of momentum generated by assisting muscle groups. For example, you may lift much more weight in a back-swinging, cheat barbell curl than in a back-straight, strict barbell curl. However, in the first technique, most of the movement force comes from the hip extensor and trunk extensor muscles. Conversely, in the second technique, most of the movement force is produced by the biceps, which is the primary purpose of performing barbell curls.

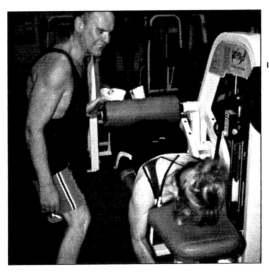

Slow training has been found to be a very effective method for accomplishing the primary purpose of high-intensity strength training, which is to make each exercise set more challenging to your target muscles.

Super-Slow® Training

During the 1980s, Ken Hutchins developed a strength training technique that extended each exercise repetition to 14 seconds. This procedure, called super-slow® training, requires 10 seconds for each lifting movement and four seconds for each lowering movement. To keep the exercise set within the time parameters of an individual's anaerobic energy system (90 seconds), only four to six repetitions are performed.

Basically, super-slow® training provides more time in the more challenging concentric (lifting) muscle actions than standard-speed training. Consider the fact that a 10-repetition set of standard-speed training (two seconds lifting, four seconds lowering) involves about 20 seconds of concentric muscle tension (10 reps x 2 seconds lifting phase). However, a 5-repetition set of super-slow training involves about 50 seconds of concentric muscle tension (5 reps x 10 seconds lifting phase). This procedure clearly makes the exercise set more difficult to perform, and typically requires less resistance than momentum-assisted training procedures.

Anyone who tries to exercise in a super-slow® manner quickly realizes that this is a very tough and tedious training technique. If you have never experienced slow-speed exercise, try doing a 14-second squat using just your bodyweight. That is, take four seconds to lower yourself from a standing position until your thighs are parallel to the floor. Now, rise, taking 10 full seconds to return to a standing position. You should feel a distinctly different and demanding effort in your quadriceps and hamstring muscles as you perform the slow upward movement (concentric muscle action). You should also understand why a single set of four to six super-slow® repetitions is sufficient to achieve a high level of muscle fatigue and strength-building stimulus.

While the level of physical discomfort is not always a reliable indicator of exercise productivity, super-slow® training has proven to be very effective for enhanced muscle conditioning. In fact, our research has shown highly significant strength gains in both beginning and advanced subjects using this exercise procedure.

Research on Super-Slow® Training

Our studies on super-slow® training were conducted under close supervision to ensure that the participants performed the 14-second repetitions properly. To maintain focus and prevent distraction from exercisers using standard training technique, our beginning subjects trained in small classes in a separate research facility. Our advanced subjects were supervised by personal trainers and served as their own control group. In this regard, they performed some exercises with super-slow® technique (specific muscle groups) and other exercises with standard technique (unrelated muscle groups). A comparison was then made between the strength gains produced by the different training procedures, assuming that muscle responsiveness is similar in most major muscle groups.

Beginning Subjects

Our first study with beginning participants involved 74 men and women who performed 13 Nautilus exercises, three days a week, for a period of eight weeks. The super-slow training group (35 subjects) did one set of four to six repetitions at 14 seconds each (10 seconds lifting, four seconds lowering). The standard training group (39 subjects) did one set of eight to 12 repetitions at seven seconds each (two seconds lifting, one second pause, four seconds lowering). It should be noted that both training protocols required the same time to complete the exercise set (5 repetitions x 14 seconds each = 70 seconds; 10 repetitions x 7 seconds each = 70 seconds).

As presented in Figure 5.2, the super-slow® training group experienced a 26.5-pound increase in their five-repetition maximum (5 RM) weightloads, whereas the standard training group experienced a 17.5-pound increase in their 10-repetition maximum (10 RM) weightloads. The results indicate that the slow-speed exercisers attained 50 percent greater strength gains (tested at slow speed) than the standard speed exercisers (tested at standard speed).

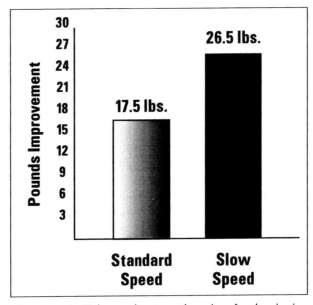

Figure 5.2 Eight-week strength gains for beginning subjects using standard-speed and slow-speed training (N = 74)

Our second study with beginning participants was essentially a replication of our first study. The 73 previously untrained participants performed 13 Nautilus exercises, two or three days a week, for a period of 10 weeks. The super-slow® training group (30 subjects) did one set of four to six repetitions at 14 seconds each (10 seconds lifting, four seconds lowering). The standard training group (43 subjects) did one set of eight to 12 repetitions (two seconds lifting, one second pause, four seconds lowering). Again, all of the study participants performed their exercise sets in essentially the same time frame (about 70 seconds each).

As illustrated in Figure 5.3, the super-slow® training group increased their 5 RM chest press weightload by 24.0 pounds, whereas the standard training group increased their 10 RM chest press weightload by 16.3 pounds. These results were almost identical to those in the first study, as the slow-speed exercisers again attained 50-percent greater strength gains (tested at slow speed) than the standard-speed exercisers (tested at standard speed).

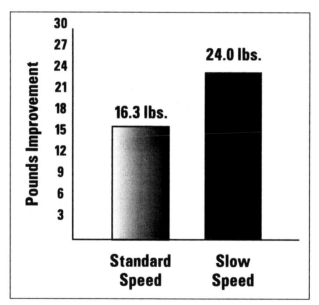

Figure 5.3 Ten-week strength gains for beginning subjects using standard-speed and slow-speed training (N = 73)

The findings from these studies with 147 new exercisers clearly indicate that super-slow® training produces a faster rate of strength development than standard training in beginning participants. As a consequence, the super-slow exercise procedure for individuals who want to gain strength more quickly during their initial training period is recommended.

Advanced Subjects

We also conducted research on super-slow® training with advanced exercisers. One study involved a comparison of two methods of slow-speed training with standard training. The 15 participants performed slow, positive-emphasis training on three exercises (leg extension, biceps curl, chin-up), slow, negative-emphasis training on three exercises (leg curl, triceps extension, bar dip), and standard training on two exercises (abdominal curl, low back extension).

Slow, positive-emphasis training consisted of performing one set of four to six repetitions at 14 seconds each, with 10 seconds for the lifting phase and four seconds for the lowering phase. Slow, negative-emphasis training consisted of doing one set of four to six repetitions at 14 seconds each, with four seconds for the lifting phase and 10 seconds for the lowering phase. Standard training consisted of engaging in one set of eight to 12 repetitions at seven seconds each (two seconds lifting, one second pause, four seconds lowering). In this manner, all of the training protocols required about the same training duration (approximately 70 seconds per set).

All of the subjects trained twice a week under careful supervision for a period of six weeks. The exercises performed with standard training increased by an average of 12 pounds. On the other hand, the exercises performed with slow positive-emphasis training increased by an average of 22 pounds, while the exercises performed with slow negative-emphasis training increased by an average of 26 pounds (see Figure 5.4). Both of the slow-speed training techniques (slow, positive-emphasis and slow, negative-emphasis) proved highly effective for these advanced exercisers. In fact, the average strength gain attained by the two slow-speed methods (24 pounds) was twice that achieved by standard-speed training (12 pounds).

In another study with already physically fit individuals, 12 men and women did super-slow strength training twice a week for a period of six weeks. The subjects in this study completed four to six repetitions of the following exercises, taking 10 seconds for each lifting movement and four seconds for each lowering movement:

- leg curl
- leg press
- chest cross
- chest press
- pullover
- pulldown

- lateral raise
- shoulder press
- biceps curl
- triceps extension
- abdominal curl
- low back extension

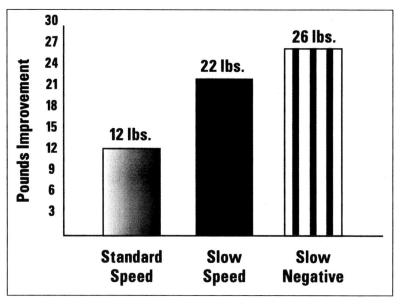

Figure 5.4 Six-week strength gains for advanced subjects using standard-speed, slow positive-emphasis, and slow negative-emphasis training (N=15)

As presented in Table 5.1, the trainees significantly increased their previous best performances in both weightstack exercises (which they did each workout) and bodyweight exercises (which they did not perform during the study period). These results provide further evidence to support super-slow® training as a productive procedure for overcoming strength plateaus.

Table 5.1 Six-week performance improvements for advanced subjects using super-slow® training (N = 12)

Lateral Raise Weightload	Chin-Ups	Bar-Dips
+ 11.0 lb	+ 1.3 reps	+ 3.0 reps
(43.3 lbs - 54.3 lbs)	(4.0 reps - 5.3 reps)	(9.0 reps - 12.0 reps)

Super-Slow® Training Considerations

Super-slow® training offers one of the simplest means for experiencing a high-intensity exercise set. Extending each repetition enhances the strength-building stimulus by increasing both muscle tension and force output. Although tedious to perform, super-slow® training can be a productive procedure for beginning and advanced participants who desire a faster rate of strength development.

• Counting Seconds

Proper performance of super-slow® training may be facilitated by having an instructor count the seconds out loud as you adjust to the new movement pattern. At first, most people move much too quickly, and their attempts to slow down typically result in ratcheted stop-and-go actions. Once you smooth-out the 10-second lifting movements, try to keep every repetition consistent by counting for yourself, using a one-thousand-one, one-thousand-two, one-thousand-three cadence.

• Breathing

After the correct movement pattern is established, work on your breathing. As you are aware, the general breathing guideline in standard training is to exhale during lifting movements and to inhale during lowering movements. However, it is unlikely you can exhale thoughout a demanding 10-second lifting action. In fact, the high-energy requirements of super-slow® exercise may require a faster breathing rate than standard training. Accordingly, it is recommended that you inhale and exhale as needed, making sure that you never hold your breath. If you prefer a more precise breathing pattern, try inhaling for two counts (one-thousand-one, one-thousand-two) and exhaling for two counts (one-thousand-three, and one-thousand-four).

• Repetitions

Individuals who are accustomed to performing eight to 12 repetitions per set may feel compelled to do so when training in a super-slow® manner. However, if you are doing more than six super-slow® repetitions, you are probably using too little resistance. For best strength gains, each set of super-slow exercise should be completed within the maximal range of your anaerobic energy system (90 seconds). Similar to eight to 12 repetitions of standard training, four to six repetitions of super-slow® training should take between 56 and 84 seconds.

• Resistance

Another problem with slower repetitions is determining the appropriate exercise weightload. Due to the reduced role of momentum, you will undoubtedly need to use less resistance for super-slow® training than for standard training, at least during the first few workouts. When you finally find weightloads that fatigue the target muscles in four to six repetitions, you should make progress at a relatively fast rate. On average, our research subjects increased their exercise weightloads by more than three pounds per week over a 6- to 10-week training period. This high rate of strength progression certainly supports the efficiency and effectiveness of super-slow® training.

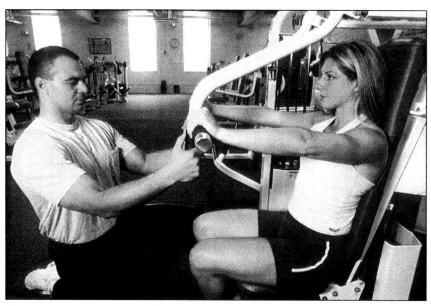

Slower movement speeds produce more muscle tension and greater muscle force.

• Periodization

Because the slow-exercise technique is demanding physically and mentally, performing six- to 12-week training periods, alternating with doing six to 12 weeks of standard training, is recommended. Although some individuals do super-slow training exclusively, periodically changing the exercise protocol reduces the risk of both staleness and burnout.

• Sample Workout

Table 5.2 presents a sample first-time super-slow workout for a person experienced in standard strength training. Suggested super-slow exercise weightloads are provided, based on the trainee's standard workout weightloads. Generally speaking, the level of resistance used in standard training is reduced about 20 percent for the initial super-slow® exercise session.

Table 5.2 An example of an initial super-slow workout with suggested exercise weightloads, based on standard training weightloads

Sample Exercises	Muscle Groups	Present Weightload for Standard Training	Initial Weightload for Super-Slow® Training
Leg Curl	Hamstrings	125 lbs x 8-12 reps	100 lbs x 4-6 reps
Leg Extension	Quadriceps	150 lbs x 8-12 reps	120 lbs x 4-6 reps
Chest Cross	Pectoralis Major	125 lbs x 8-12 reps	100 lbs x 4-6 reps
Pullover	Latissimus Dorsi	200 lbs x 8-12 reps	160 lbs x 4-6 reps
Lateral Raise	Deltoids	100 lbs x 8-12 reps	80 lbs x 4-6 reps
Biceps Curl	Biceps	75 lbs x 8-12 reps	60 lbs x 4-6 reps
Triceps Extension	Triceps	75 lbs x 8-12 reps	60 lbs x 4-6 reps
Low Back	Erector Spinae	140 lbs x 8-12 reps	110 lbs x 4-6 reps
Abdominal	Rectus Abdominis	140 lbs x 8-12 reps	110 lbs x 4-6 reps
Neck Flexion	Neck Flexors	115 lbs x 8-12 reps	90 lbs x 4-6 reps
Neck Extension	Neck Extensors	150 lbs x 8-12 reps	120 lbs x 4-6 reps

* Note: When seven repetitions can be properly performed, the exercise resistance is increased by five percent or less.

6

Combined Training Program

In previous chapters, the following different high-intensity training techniques that have proven to be more effective than standard training for enhancing muscle strength in beginning and advanced exercisers were reviewed:

- *Breakdown training* that extends the exercise set by reducing the resistance and performing a few post-fatigue repetitions.

- *Assisted training* that extends the exercise set by receiving help from a partner (lifting movements only) for a few post-fatigue repetitions.

- *Pre-exhaustion training* that extends the exercise set by performing two successive exercises (rotary followed by linear) for the target muscle group.

- *Slow positive-emphasis training* that extends the exercise repetition with a 10-second lifting movement and a four-second lowering movement.

- *Slow negative-emphasis training* that extends the exercise repetition with a four-second lifting movement and a 10-second lowering movement.

While several other advanced-training procedures exist, these five high-intensity techniques are recommended because they offer a relatively low risk of injury and a relatively high rate of strength development. These five exercise procedures are also very time-efficient, making them particularly practical and attractive to those individuals who have limited time to train. In our opinion, all three factors (low risk of injury, high rate of productivity, time efficiency) are essential elements of a safe, successful and sensible strength training protocol.

Because variety is an important program component for achieving and maintaining continual progress, adding all five of these exercise tools to your strength-training toolbox can be very beneficial. You can actually combine different high-intensity techniques into a one- or two-month program that can heighten the demands placed on your muscular system, while also maintaining your level of mental freshness. In this regard, we have had excellent experiences with our six-week combined training program, particularly with respect to participant response and results.

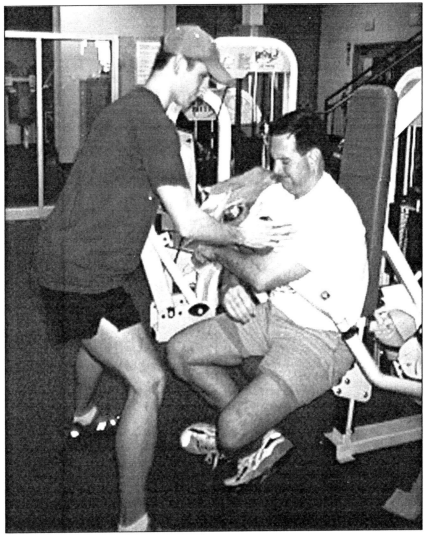

Variety is an important component for achieving and maintaining continual progress from your strength-training efforts.

Six-Week Combined Training Program

Over the years, we have conducted several strength-training studies of varying durations, typically between four and 14 weeks. Although a legitimate argument can be made for longer research programs, we have found that six weeks of high-intensity workouts are well-received by our participants. While four-week programs may be too brief to attain maximum strength gains, eight-week programs may be too long to maintain optimum participant motivation.

Our six-week combined training program involves one week of each high-intensity exercise technique, followed by an idividual's preferred procedure during the final week. As presented in Table 6.1, breakdown training is performed during the first week, assisted training in the second week, slow positive-emphasis training in the third week, slow negative-emphasis training in the fourth week, pre-exhaustion training in the fifth week, and the high-intensity technique that a person felt was most productive for that individual is repeated during the sixth week.

Table 6.1 An example of a combined high-intensity training program including weeks, days, techniques, exercises, and time requirements

Weeks	Days	High-Intensity Training Technique	Total Exercises	Total Time
1	Monday and Friday	Breakdown Training (10 reps to fatigue; 3 reps with 10%-20% less weight)	10-12	20-24 Minutes
2	Monday and Friday	Assisted Training (10 reps to fatigue; 3 reps with partner assistance on lifting phase)	10-12	20-24 Minutes
3	Monday and Friday	Slow Positive-Emphasis Training (5 reps to fatigue; 10 seconds lifting and 4 seconds lowering)	10-12	20-24 Minutes
4	Monday and Friday	Slow Negative-Emphasis Training (5 reps to fatigue; 4 seconds lifting and 10 seconds lowering)	10-12	20-24 Minutes
5	Monday and Friday	Pre-Exhaustion Training (10 reps to fatigue followed by 5 reps with second exercise)	14-16	24-28 Minutes
6	Monday and Friday	Personal Preference (Trainee chooses favorite high-intensity technique)	10-16	20-28 Minutes

Although the specific high-intensity program employed may be varied from session to session, the twelve exercise stations typically used for breakdown, assisted, and super-slow® training are as follows: leg extension; leg curl; hip adduction; hip abduction; chest cross, pullover; lateral raise; biceps curl; triceps extension; low back extension; abdominal curl; and neck. Likewise, the sixteen exercise stations employed for pre-exhaustion training are as follows: leg extension; leg press; leg curl; hip extension; chest cross; chest press; pullover; pulldown; lateral raise; shoulder press; biceps curl; assisted chin-up; triceps extension; assisted bar-dip; low back extension; and abdominal curl. It should be noted these exercised are paired with a rotary exercise, followed by a linear exercise for each target muscle group. Of course, the training protocol may be altered as desired as long as the program addresses all of the major muscle groups.

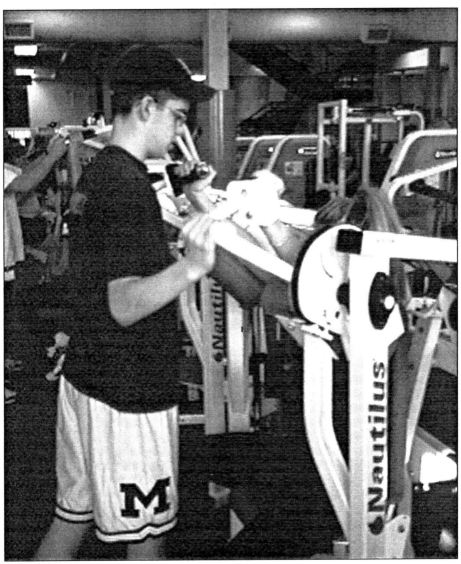

Different high-intensity training techniques can be combined into a one- or two-month program that can heighten the demands placed on your muscular system.

Combined Training Program Research

We recently studied the effects of our combined high-intensity training program on the level of muscle strength and body composition of 48 advanced participants who followed the exercise protocol presented in Table 6.1. All of the subjects worked with a personal trainer during their scheduled exercise sessions. No subject received nutritional information or dietary guidelines during the study, so our only intervention was the combined high-intensity training sessions.

After six weeks incorporating all of the high-intensity exercise techniques, the subjects experienced significant improvements in their level of muscle strength and body composition. As shown in Figure 6.1, the participants increased their average

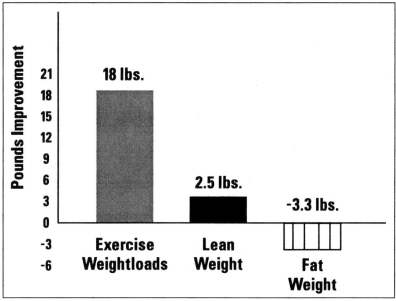

Figure 6.1 Six-week changes in exercise weightloads, lean weight and fat weight for intermediate level subjects using the combined high-intensity training program (N=48)

exercise weightloads by 18 pounds. They also added 2.5 pounds of lean (muscle) weight and lost 3.3 pounds of fat weight, for a six-pound change in body composition. Stated differently, the 48 intermediate trainees gained strength at the rate of three pounds per week and improved their body composition at the rate of one pound per week.

Concluding Comments

Excellent results have been achieved from performing a combined high-intensity exercise program that includes one week each of breakdown, assisted, pre-exhaustion, slow positive-emphasis and slow negative-emphasis training, plus a week of the individual's preferred training technique. Our research on 48 intermediate level men and women who followed this training protocol, using 12 to 16 machine exercises for a period of six weeks, revealed an average strength increase of 18 pounds, an average muscle gain of 2.5 pounds, and an average fat loss of 3.3 pounds. These results represent a high rate of strength gain and body composition improvement for experienced subjects, which should be very encouraging news for those exercisers who want to surpass a training plateau.

Because all of the high-intensity training techniques are physically demanding and mentally challenging, the combined program provides a variety of exercise procedures that reduces the risk of overtraining and burnout. By changing the training protocol every two-exercise sessions, the participants tend to maintain a fresh perspective and a positive attitude towards their high-intensity workouts.

Of course, the five basic procedures for extending the exercise set and the exercise repetition may be presented in a variety of combinations. Likewise, you may use different training durations for the exercise techniques. For example, you may prescribe a 10-week training program with two weeks of each exercise procedure. Or you may prefer a nine-week combination program that involves three weeks each of the three extended-set techniques (breakdown training, assisted training, pre-exhaustion training) without performing either of the extended-repetition techniques (slow positive-emphasis training, slow negative-emphasis training). Whatever combination of techniques you choose, the key to a successful combined training program is regular change. In other words, you should perform a few sessions of one exercise procedure, balanced with a few sessions of a different exercise procedure. This approach will result in a consistent application of all the desired training techniques.

After completing a combined high-intensity training program, you should undertake an equal period of standard exercise procedures to firmly establish your new strength level. Alternating between high-intensity and standard strength training is a simple, but effective, means for periodically enhancing your training stimulus, without exceeding reasonable physical and mental parameters.

7

Combined Exercise Protocol

We recently designed a high-intensity training program that incorporated a combined-exercise protocol. The primary objective of our efforts was to identify a more challenging training approach that would provide a safe, effective, and efficient alternative to the traditional boot-camp conditioning programs universally used for military and police recruits. Although differences exist between the various boot-camp conditioning programs, these regimes typically emphasize lots of running and almost unlimited repetitions of bodyweight exercises, such as push-ups, sit-ups, and squat thrusts.

Boot Camp Training

Boot camp training has a long history of success for short-term conditioning, and offers certain practical advantages over standard strength-training programs. Among the advantages of boot-camp training are no required exercise facilities, no required exercise equipment, and only one instructor for a large number of trainees.

Unfortunately, traditional boot-camp programs suffer from two weaknesses, both of which have become more problematic during the past several years. The first potential weakness involves a "physical" concern. Boot-camp training can lead to a variety of overuse injuries, resulting from repetitive movement patterns of calisthenics exercises that place high stress on the musculoskeletal system.

The second possible limitation involves a "mental" concern. Boot-camp training may result in burnout that arises from performing seemingly endless repetitions of the same calisthenics exercises. The burnout factor appears to have particularly long-lasting effects, as evidenced by the many military and police recruits who stop exercising completely at the conclusion of their boot-camp training program.

Standard Strength Training

Standard strength training uses free-weights or machines to provide progressive resistance exercise that offers more muscle-building stimulus than fixed resistance exercise performed with bodyweight. Unfortunately, standard strength training typically requires designated exercise facilities, specialized exercise equipment, small conditioning classes, longer workout sessions, and a longer time frame for fitness development. As a result, these factors have rendered standard strength training less feasible than boot-camp exercise for most military and police conditioning environments.

High-Intensity Strength Training

As you have discovered in the proceeding chapters of this book, high-intensity strength training has two very distinct advantages over standard programs of strength exercise. First, high-intensity workouts are more time-efficient, typically requiring less than 30 minutes for completion. Second, high-intensity exercise procedures are more productive, generally resulting in greater strength and muscle gains during a given training period.

With these benefits in mind, we recently conducted a research study to compare the results of a high-intensity strength training program with a boot-camp conditioning program. To maximize training effectiveness and efficiency, we combined two of the high-intensity procedures and used relatively high exercise weightloads. We refer to this program as the combined exercise protocol.

Combined Exercise Protocol

Our combined exercise protocol represents the most challenging, high-intensity training program that we have researched to date. To generate significant strength gains within a brief conditioning period (five weeks), we incorporated a higher percentage of maximum resistance than is normally used.

Most high-intensity training techniques (breakdown, assisted, pre-exhaustion) are performed with the eight to 10-repetition maximum (8-10 RM) weightload, which corresponds to about 75 to 80 percent of the heaviest resistance possible for a single repetition. However, in this study, we increased the work effort by using the subjects' five-repetition maximum (5 RM) weightload for most of the training exercises. The 5 RM weightload represents about 85 to 90 percent of the heaviest resistance possible for a single repetition.

Several of the training exercises were performed in a pre-exhaustion sequence to further enhance the strength-building stimulus. As was discussed previously, pre-exhaustion training involves performing essentially two successive sets of two different exercises for the same target muscle. The first exercise is a rotary movement to isolate and fatigue the target muscle. This exercise is followed as quickly as possible by a linear movement exercise that incorporates a fresh assisting muscle to further fatigue the target muscle.

For example, to facilitate chest development, we paired the chest cross (rotary) and chest press (linear) exercises. To facilitate upper back development, the pullover (rotary) and seated row (linear) exercises were paired. To facilitate shoulder development, we paired the lateral raise (rotary) and shoulder press (linear) exercises. In each combination, the second exercise incorporated fresh arm muscles to force the pre-fatigued torso muscles to work longer and harder, thereby attaining a greater

Table 7.1 Exercise sequence, target muscles, training resistance and repetitions scheme for first combined high-intensity exercise protocol

Exercise	Target Muscle	Training Resistance	Repetitions Scheme*
Leg Extension	Quadriceps	5 RM	5 reps + 5 assists
Leg Curl	Hamstrings	5 RM	5 reps + 5 assists
Leg Press	Quadriceps Hamstrings	5 RM	5 reps + 5 assists
Chest Cross	Pectoralis Major	5 RM	5 reps + 5 assists
Chest Press	Pectoralis Major Triceps	5 RM	5 reps + 5 assists
Pullover	Latissimus Dorsi	5 RM	5 reps + 5 assists
Seated Row	Latissimus Dorsi Biceps	5 RM	5 reps + 5 assists
Lateral Raise	Deltoids	5 RM	5 reps + 5 assists
Shoulder Press	Deltoids Triceps	5 RM	5 reps + 5 assists
Biceps Curl	Biceps	5 RM	5 reps + 5 assists
Triceps Extension	Triceps	5 RM	5 reps + 5 assists
Abdominal Curl	Rectus Abdominis	5 RM	5 reps + 5 assists
Low Back Extension	Erector Spinae	10 RM	10 reps + no assists

*Note: When six repetitions can be properly performed, the exercise resistance is increased by five percent or less.

training effect. Table 7-1 presents the exercise sequence, target muscles, training resistance, and repetitions scheme used in this study.

In addition to relatively heavy weightloads and pre-exhaustion exercises, the combined high-intensity protocol features assisted training to assure a high level of both concentric and eccentric muscle fatigue. As was discussed previously, this technique uses an assistant to help lift the resistance when your muscles become too fatigued to do so. The assistant provides just enough help to lift the weightstack five more times. Of course, each successive repetition requires more assistance due to progressive fatigue in your target muscles.

Because muscles are approximately 40 percent stronger in lowering (eccentric) actions than lifting (concentric) actions, the assistant helps on the lifting movements only. However, as the target muscles fatigue, controlled lowering movements become more demanding and provide additional stimulus for strength development.

The combination of 5 RM training weightloads, pre-exhaustion exercise sequences, and five post-fatigue assisted repetitions forces the muscles to work much harder than standard workouts, resulting in greater strength gains, as long as sufficient recovery and building time is provided. In order to ensure that your body has sufficient time to both build and recover, it is recommended that you only do two combined exercise protocol training sessions per week.

Research Study

In our initial study that investigated the effects of performing a combined exercise protocol, 29 previously trained and well-conditioned adults (20 males and 9 females, mean age 35 years) completed five weeks of advanced workouts. All of the participants performed at least one bodyweight chin-up (range one to 20) and at least one bodyweight bar dip (range one to 33) in their pre-training assessments.

Five subjects did 10 one-hour boot-camp workouts (on Mondays and Fridays), consisting of various calisthenics and bodyweight exercises, conducted by the trainer for the Massachusetts Police Academy recruits. Twenty-four subjects did 10 half-hour combined exercise protocol high-intensity strength training sessions (on Mondays and Fridays), conducted by experienced personal trainers.

As presented in Table 7.1, the high-intensity trainees performed the low back extension exercise for one set, using the 10 RM weightload. Because this particular exercise involves potential vulnerable aspects of the spinal column, it was done in the standard manner. Each subject performed the leg extension, leg curl, leg press, chest cross, chest press, pullover, seated row, lateral raise, shoulder press, biceps curl, and triceps extension exercises for one set each, using the 5 RM weightload. When the subjects reached a point of muscle fatigue in these exercises, an assistant helped on the lifting phase of five additional repetitions. Every repetition, pre-fatigue and post-fatigue, was completed in about six seconds, with two seconds for the lifting movement and four seconds for the lowering movement.

The effects of the boot camp and the combined exercise protocol were evaluated by the increase in bodyweight chin-ups and bar-dips, as assessed before and after the five-week training period. To avoid testing bias, the subjects did not perform chin-ups or bar-dips in either training program, and promised not to do these exercises at any time during the research period.

As shown in Table 7.2, the boot-camp participants averaged 1.2 more chin-ups and 2.8 more bar-dips after completing their training program. The high-intensity trainees averaged 2.0 more chin-ups and 4.2 more bar-dips after their training program. As another indicator of strength improvement, the high-intensity group increased their 5 RM weightload by 31.4 pounds in the leg extension exercise and by 17.5 pounds in the lateral raise exercise. All of the performance improvements attained by the combined exercise protocol participants were statistically significant ($p < 0.05$). In addition, psychological assessments administered before and after the training program showed no signs of mental burnout in the high-intensity exercise group. Unfortunately, the small number of subjects in the boot-camp training program precluded meaningful statistical analyses.

Table 7.2 Five-week results for experienced subjects using either boot-camp training or first high-intensity combined exercise protocol (N = 29)

	N	Age (Yrs)	Chin-Ups (Reps)	Bar-Dips (Reps)	Leg Ext (Lbs)	Lateral Raise (Lbs)
Boot Camp	5	35.4	+1.2 (6.4 - 7.6)	+2.8 (11.6 - 14.4)		
High-Intensity	24	34.9	+2.0 (5.6 - 7.6)	+4.2 (9.8 - 14.0)	+31.4 (149.5 - 180.9)	+17.5 (104.8 - 122.3)

Despite the inability to do a useful statistical analysis of the efforts of the boot-camp subjects, the results of this study confirm that traditional boot-camp workouts are effective for improving physical performance in bodyweight exercises, such as chin-ups and bar-dips. The findings further demonstrate that 30-minute high-intensity training sessions compare favorably with 60-minute, boot-camp workouts. In fact, two relatively brief weekly workouts, using the combined-exercise protocol, produced impressive improvements in chin-up, bar-dip, leg extension, and lateral raise performance after just five weeks of training.

It would appear that the combined high-intensity exercise protocol offers several advantages over traditional boot-camp conditioning classes. These differences are addressed in Table 7.3.

Table 7.3 Advantages of the combined high-intensity exercise protocol over traditional boot-camp training

Considerations	High Intensity Training	Boot Camp Training
Progressive resistance	Yes	No
Session duration	Short	Long
Instructor assistance	Yes	No
Rate of strength development	Faster	Slower
Risk of overuse injury	Lower	Higher
Risk of mental burnout	Lower	Higher

Follow-up Research Study

We subsequently conducted a follow-up study to see if similar results could be attained by training with a lower percentage of maximum resistance. Instead of using the subjects' 5 RM weightload (85 to 90 percent of maximum resistance), we incorporated the subjects' 8 RM weightload (75 to 80 percent of maximum resistance). The 15 well-conditioned subjects in this study followed essentially the same high-intensity strength training protocol used in the previous research program, with one major difference. Instead of doing five repetitions to fatigue, followed by five assisted repetitions, this training group performed eight repetitions to fatigue, followed by four assisted repetitions (see Table 7.4).

Although this protocol represented a somewhat less-intense training protocol (more repetitons with relatively less resistance), the results were very similar to those in the first study. As presented in Table 7.5, these trainees averaged 1.4 more chin-ups and 4.5 more bar dips after completing their exercise program. They also increased their 8 RM leg extension weightload by 30.0 pounds and their 8 RM lateral raise weightload by 10.6 pounds. In addition, they improved their body composition level from 22.7 percent fat to 21.5 percent fat, as assessed with skinfold measurements. All of the pre-training to post-training changes were statistically significant ($p < 0.05$).

Table 7.4 Exercise sequence, target muscles, training resistance and repetitions scheme for second combined high-intensity exercise protocol

Exercise	Target Muscle	Training Resistance	Repetitions Scheme*
Leg Extension	Quadriceps	8 RM	8 reps + 4 assists
Leg Curl	Hamstrings	8 RM	8 reps + 4 assists
Leg Press	Quadriceps Hamstrings	8 RM	8 reps + 4 assists
Chest Cross	Pectoralis Major	8 RM	8 reps + 4 assists
Chest Press	Pectoralis Major Triceps	8 RM	8 reps + 4 assists
Pullover	Latissimus Dorsi	8 RM	8 reps + 4 assists
Pulldown	Latissimus Dorsi Biceps	8 RM	8 reps + 4 assists
Lateral Raise	Deltoids	8 RM	8 reps + 4 assists
Shoulder Press	Deltoids Triceps	8 RM	8 reps + 4 assists
Biceps Curl	Biceps	8 RM	8 reps + 4 assists
Triceps Extension	Triceps	8 RM	8 reps + 4 assists
Abdominal Curl	Rectus Abdominis	8 RM	8 reps + 4 assists
Low Back Extension	Erector Spinae	8 RM	8 reps + 4 assists

*Note: When nine repetitions can be properly performed the exercise resistance is increased by five percent or less.

Table 7.5 Five-week results for experienced subjects, using a second high-intensity combined exercise protocol (N = 15)

N	Age (Yrs)	Chin-Ups Reps	Bar-Dips Reps	Lbs	Lbs	Fat %
15	37.8	+1.4 (4.7 - 6.1)	+4.5 (9.6 - 14.1)	30.0 (120.5 - 150.5)	+10.6 (66.2 - 76.8)	-1.2 (22.7 - 21.5)

Physical abilities were different in the two high-intensity training groups due to the higher ratio of men to women in the first study. To more accurately compare the training effects of the two exercise protocols, we examined the percentage improvements in all of the performance categories. As shown in Table 7.6, the percentage improvements were very close for both high-intensity strength training programs. These results indicate that doing five repetitions followed by five assists and doing eight repetitions followed by four assists produces similar strength improvements. Although no injuries were reported in either of the study groups, eight repetitions, followed by four assists seems to be a safer training protocol due to lower resistance levels. Accordingly, it is recommended that you use the more conservative 8 RM exercise weightload for eight good repetitions, followed by four assisted repetitions for first-time participants.

Table 7.6 Percentage improvements for strength parameters in two high-intensity combined exercise protocols (N = 39)

Training Program	Chin-Up (Reps)	Bar-Dip (Reps)	Leg Ext (Lbs)	Lat Raise (Lbs)
5 Reps + 5 Assists	+36%	+43%	+21%	+17%
8 Reps + 4 Assists	+30%	+47%	+25%	+16%

Although this high-intensity strength training protocol is physically demanding, each exercise is performed for only one set of 12 repetitions. As a consequence, we have experienced no problems with either muscle overuse injuries or mental burnout. For logistical purposes, the combined exercise protocol may be conducted with one or two instructors and with up to 30 participants working as partners in the manner detailed in the next section of this chapter.

Group Training Design

- Select 15 resistance machines that provide a comprehensive workout for all the major muscle groups.

- Have one or two qualified instructors teach the training techniques and supervise each exercise session.

- Pair trainees at each machine, thereby accommodating up to 30 participants per session.

- Designate one partner as the exerciser and one partner as the assistant.

- Have the exercisers complete the 15-machine circuit in 30 minutes by rotating stations every two minutes.

- Have the exercisers perform about eight repetitions to muscle fatigue with the 8 RM weightload.

- Have the assistants provide manual assistance on four post-fatigue repetitions (lifting phase only) on the designated exercises.

- At the completion of the workout, reverse roles and have the new assistants take the new exercisers through the circuit.

Concluding Comments

Although the group-training protocol reviewed in this chapter requires one hour for completion, each participant performs only 30 minutes of high-intensity strength training. In fact, the actual exercise time is about 18 minutes (15 exercises at 72 seconds each). As such, this training protocol represents a highly efficient and effective means of strength-building that can accommodate a relatively large number of exercisers. The evidence is compelling that the combined high-intensity exercise program provides an advantageous alternative to traditional boot-camp training, both physiologically and psychologically. It offers a higher rate of strength development, a lower risk of overuse injuries, and less potential for mental burnout.

8

Using the Right
Repetition Range

The proceeding chapters of this book have presented several high-intensity training techniques for extending the exercise set and exercise repetition in order to more effectively fatigue the target muscles and enhance strength development. Various training programs have also been reviewed that combine different high-intensity exercise procedures into more challenging workouts for even greater strength gains. This chapter is intended to provide additional information on repetition ranges that should further facilitate positive muscle response to your high-intensity strength training program.

Understanding Repetition Ranges

As a rule, when you engage in strength exercise, it is recommended that you use an initial resistance level that fatigues the target muscle within eight to 12 repetitions for breakdown, assisted and pre-exhaustion training, and a weightload that fatigues the target muscle within four to six repetitions for super-slow training. As was previously discussed, all of these exercise techniques are designed to cause muscle fatigue within time parameters imposed by your anaerobic energy system, typically between 50 and 75 seconds.

Reaching muscle fatigue within 50 to 75 seconds is ideal for most individuals, but not for everyone. The vast majority of individuals have a fairly even mix of fast-twitch and slow-twitch muscle fibers, which collectively produce high levels of muscle force for about 50 to 75 seconds. This time frame involves the normal range of your body's anaerobic energy system.

However, a small percentage of the population are born with a high ratio of fast-twitch to slow-twitch muscle fibers, giving them a shorter period of high-force muscle production. This situation occurs because fast-twitch fibers fatigue faster than slow-twitch fibers, resulting in relatively brief bouts of high-effort exercise. As such, these individuals have low-endurance muscles.

For example, a person with predominately fast-twitch muscle fibers may have a high-force production capacity of only 25 to 50 seconds. This individual would not be well-served with a training set that lasted 75 seconds, because the exercise resistance would necessarily be too light to offer an optimum strength-building stimulus. For trainees with low-endurance muscles, performing sets of four to eight repetitions is far more productive than doing sets of eight to 12 repetitions, due to better matching of exercise duration and muscle physiology.

On the other side of the same coin, a small percentage of the population exists who are born with a high ratio of slow-twitch to fast-twitch muscle fibers, giving them a longer period of high-force muscle production. This trait occurs because slow-twitch fibers fatigue slower than fast-twitch fibers, resulting in relatively long bouts of high-effort exercise. As such, these individuals have high-endurance muscles.

For example, a person with predominantly slow-twitch muscle fibers may have a high-force production capacity of 75 to 100 seconds. Such an individual would not be well-served with a training set that lasted 50 seconds, because the exercise duration would necessarily be too short for an optimum strength-building stimulus. For trainees with high-endurance muscles, sets of 12 to 16 repetitions are more productive than sets of eight to 12 repetitions due to better matching of exercise duration and muscle physiology.

Putting these principles into practice is essential for competitive athletes who participate in high-power or high-endurance sports events. Top sprinters, who typically have about 85 percent fast-twitch fibers in their quadriceps muscles, respond better to low-repetition training. This factor is also true for professional football players, who generally perform four to eight repetitions per set in their strength workouts.

Conversely, top marathon runners, who typically have about 90 percent slow-twitch muscle fibers in their quadriceps muscles, respond better to high-repetition training. This reality is equally true for elite triathletes, who should perform as many as 15 to 20 repetitions in each set of strength exercise.

Assessing Your Muscle Endurance

While you may find this information both interesting and important, it is not very practical unless you have a simple means for assessing your level of general muscle endurance. Of course, you can simply look at your personal sports performance, but this approach is unlikely to provide precise training guidelines. For example, if you are a successful power athlete, you probably have more fast-twitch muscle fibers, and if you are a successful endurance athlete, you probably have more slow-twitch muscle fibers. However, such knowledge is usually insufficient to establish a specific repetition range for attaining optimum strength development.

A more precise approach for determining your position on the power-endurance continuum is the standard vertical jump test. How high you can jump from a standing, two-foot take-off is a good indicator of your power production. Nonetheless, it does not provide enough information to develop specific repetitions recommendations for greatest strength gains.

Research on Repetition Range Determination

Over the years, we have researched an assessment procedure that has proven reasonably predictive with respect to muscle endurance, and provides relevant repetition guidelines for maximizing your strength-building stimulus. Our research model is based on a large study in which we tested 141 men and women for muscle endurance, using 75 percent of their maximum resistance (see Figure 8.1). Although the majority of subjects were average strength-trained individuals with a relatively even mix of fast-twitch and slow-twitch muscle fibers, we included a substantial number of elite power athletes and endurance athletes (e.g., winner of the Iron Man Triathlon, runnerup in NCAA 10,000 meter run, etc.). All of the study participants had essentially the same strength training background, namely, three weekly workouts, using a single set of eight to 12 repetitions for 13 Nautilus exercises.

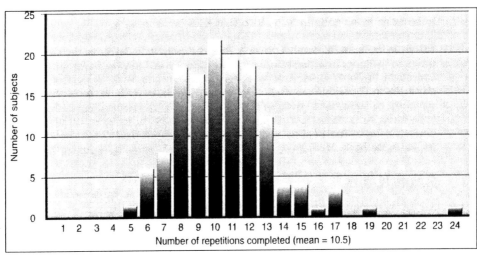

Figure 8.1

In our study, all of the subjects were assessed on the Nautilus 10-degree chest machine, a chest fly movement that addresses the pectoralis major muscles. The testing procedure that we employed involved a series of warm-up sets with progressively heavier weightloads and fewer repetitions. Typically, the assessment was initiated with about 30-percent less resistance than the subjects' 10-repetition training weightload. Ten repetitions of the exercise at this resistance level were performed. After a two-minute recovery period the participant then performed five repetitions with his/her 10-repetition training weightload. After another two-minute recovery period, the subject did a single repetition with about 30 percent more resistance than his/her 10-repetition training weightload. After another two-minute recovery period, the resistance was increased by a small amount to determine the subject's one-repetition maximum (1 RM) weightload. Generally, one to three additional trials were needed to find the heaviest resistance the participant could lift one time in perfect form. The definition of "perfect form" that was used in this situation was performing a full-range movement, with a two-second lifting phase and a four-second lowering phase.

Upon determining the individual's 1 RM weightload, that person then rested for a five-minute recovery period, while exactly 75 percent of his/her 1 RM weightload was placed on the weightstack. The subject then performed as many perfect repetitions as possible with 75 percent of the individual's maximum resistance.

Individuals who completed between eight and 12 repetitions were classified as having moderate-endurance muscles, presumably due to a relatively even mix of fast-twitch and slow-twitch muscle fibers. Those who completed fewer than eight repetitions were classified as having low-endurance muscles, presumably due to a larger percentage of fast-twitch muscle fibers. Subjects who completed more than 12 repetitions were classified as having high-endurance muscles, presumably due to a larger percentage of slow-twitch muscle fibers.

Once this information was obtained, we designed a personalized strength-training program that attempted to match the repetitions protocol to the participant's muscle physiology. As a result, we trained low-endurance individuals with fewer (4 to 8) repetitions, moderate-endurance clients with standard (8 to 12) repetitions, and high-endurance participants with more (12 to 16) repetitions (see Table 8.1). While some muscles have predominantly slow-twitch fibers (e.g., soleus), and others have predominantly fast-twitch fibers (e.g., triceps), the pectoralis major, quadriceps, and other major muscle groups normally have a pretty even mix of fiber types. Testing these muscle groups therefore provides useful information about an individual's general level of muscle endurance. In other words, if you completed only five repetitions in the chest exercise assessment, an assumption was made that all of your major muscle groups have a higher than average percentage of fast-twitch fibers. As a result, you would be encouraged to use a lower repetition protocol for all of your training exercises.

Table 8.1 Recommended time and repetitions relationships for persons with different muscle fiber characteristics

Muscle Endurance Classification	Muscle Fiber Composition	Time Per Exercise Set	Repetitions Per Exercise Set
Low-Endurance Muscles	Higher Percentage of Fast-Twitch Fibers	25-50 Seconds	4 to 8 Repetitions
Moderate-Endurance Muscles	Even Mix of Fast and Slow-Twitch Fibers	50-75 Seconds	8 to 12 Repetitions
High-Endurance Muscles	Higher Percentage of Slow-Twitch Fibers	75-100 Seconds	12 to 16 Repetitions

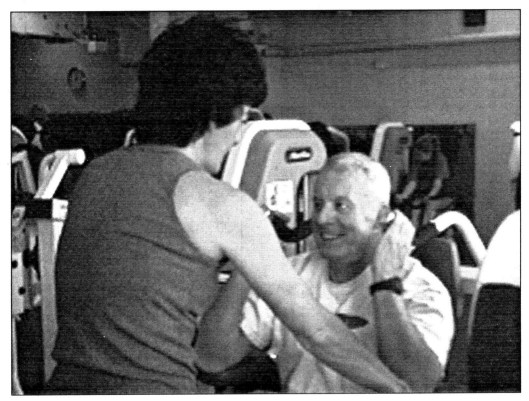

Reaching muscle fatigue within 50 to 75 seconds is ideal for most individuals, but not for everyone.

Sample Testing and Training Procedure

Consider the following example of our muscle testing and training system. Assume that Susan has been training regularly, and typically performs 10 repetitions with 70 pounds in the Nautilus 10-degree chest exercise.

Step #1   Susan performs 10 repetitions with 50 pounds on the 10-degree chest machine (first level warm-up with about 30 percent less than training resistance).

Step #2   Susan rests two minutes, then performs five repetitions with 70 pounds on on the 10-degree chest machine (second level warm-up with training resistance).

Step #3   Susan rests two minutes, then performs one repetition with 90 pounds on the 10-degree chest machine (third level warm-up with about 30 percent more than training resistance).

Step #4   Susan rests two minutes, then just barely completes one repetition with 100 pounds, which represents her maximum resistance in this exercise (1 RM).

Step #5   Susan rests five minutes, then completes 14 perfect repetitions with 75 pounds (75 percent of her 1 RM weightload).

Step #6   We classify Susan as having high-endurance muscles, presumably due to an above average percentage of slow-twitch muscle fibers.

Step #7   We suggest that Susan train with 13 to 15 repetitions to better match her exercise duration to her muscle physiology. At six seconds per repetition, she will fatigue her target muscles in about 80 to 90 seconds, which corresponds to her more enduring anaerobic energy system.

Step #8   We recommend that Susan increase her exercise resistance by five percent or less whenever she completes 15 repetitions in perfect form.

Step #9   Although higher repetitions should produce greater strength gains for Susan, we suggest that she periodically switch to a different exercise protocol (e.g., 10 to 12 repetitions) to prevent her muscles from becoming accustomed to the same training stimulus.

Research on Repetition Range Application

Understanding your muscle-endurance capacity and training in accordance with your genetic characteristics can enhance your strength development. In an attempt to learn more about the role a person's muscle endurance capacity should have on that individual's training protocol, we conducted a repetition study with 13 female track and field athletes from one of the top-ranked high school teams in New England (four-time New England cross-country champions). After assessing the young women for muscle endurance, we placed them in appropriate exercise protocols for an eight-week training period.

The power athletes (e.g., sprinters, jumpers and throwers), who tested low in muscle endurance, trained with six to eight repetitions per set. The half-milers, who tested moderate in muscle endurance, trained with nine to 11 repetitions per set. The distance runners (e.g., two milers), who tested high in muscle endurance, trained with 12 to 14 repetitions per set.

As presented in Table 8.2, the power athletes who trained with low repetitions, the half-milers who trained with moderate repetitions, and the distance runners who trained with high repetitions all experienced essentially equal gains in muscle strength. The critical point that this data illustrates is that, when the repetitions protocol is matched to the trainee's muscle endurance, excellent results may be expected, regardless of the individual's physiological characteristics.

Application to High-Intensity Training

How does your muscle endurance affect your high-intensity training program? With extended-repetition training (slow positive-emphasis or slow negative-emphasis), you simply perform fewer or more repetitions to match the exercise duration to your muscle physiology. For example, if you test low in muscle endurance, you may attain greater strength gains by training with three to four super-slow® repetitions per set (40 to 55 seconds). Conversely, if you test high in muscle endurance, you may experience better results by training with six to seven super-slow repetitions per set (85 to 100 seconds).

With extended-set training (breakdown, assisted, or pre-exhaustion), you want to complete the entire exercise (pre-fatigue and post-fatigue repetitions) within the time parameters imposed by your anaerobic energy system. As presented in the preceding chapters, if you have a relatively even muscle fiber mix, you should probably complete eight to 10 pre-fatigue repetitions (48 to 60 seconds), followed immediately by four to five post-fatigue repetitions (24 to 30 seconds) for about 72 to 90 seconds of continuous-effort resistance exercise.

However, if you test low in muscle endurance, it is probably more productive to complete six to eight pre-fatigue repetitions (36 to 48 seconds), followed immediately by three to four post-fatigue repetitions (18 to 24 seconds) for about 54 to 72 seconds of continuous muscle effort. On the other hand, if you test high in muscle endurance, you may benefit more by performing 10 to 12 pre-fatigue repetitions (60 to 72 seconds), followed immediately by five to six post-fatigue repetitions (30 to 36 seconds) for about 90 to 108 seconds of continuous-effort resistance exercise.

Table 8.2 Strength gains for track and field athletes training with specific repetition ranges (N=13)

Athletic Event	Muscle Endurance Classification	Muscle Fiber Composition	Repetition Training Range	Strength Gain 10-Degree Chest Machine
Sprints Jumps Throws	Low-Endurance Muscles	Higher Percentage of Fast-Twitch Fibers	6-8 Reps	+22.5 lbs
Half-Mile	Moderate-Endurance Muscles	Even Mix of Fast and Slow-Twitch Fibers	9-11 Reps	+21.0 lbs
Two-Mile	High-Endurance Muscles	Higher Percentage of Slow-Twitch Fibers	12-14 Reps	+20.0 lbs

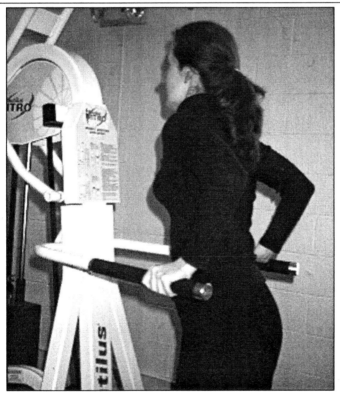

When the repetitions protocol is matched to the trainee's level of muscle endurance, excellent results may be expected, regardless of the individual's physiological considerations.

Although it might appear that higher-repetition training is more challenging than lower-repetition training, this assumption is not necessarily true. Higher-repetition training should be challenging and most productive for people with high muscle endurance, whereas lower-repetition training should be challenging and most productive for individuals with low muscle endurance. Remember that the main objective of identifying and using your personalized repetition range is to better match the exercise duration with your inherent muscle physiology.

Concluding Comments

Our research has developed a simple assessment tool for estimating your relative level of muscle endurance, which is largely based on your ratio of fast-twitch to slow-twitch muscle fibers. Because your muscle fiber make-up is a genetic characteristic that is not altered significantly through training, it makes sense to train in a manner that best matches your repetitions protocol to your muscle physiology. Accordingly, we encourage you to perform this assessment procedure, and to train in an appropriate manner in order to achieve your highest rate of strength gain.

9

Recommendations for Best Results

The high-intensity exercise techniques and training programs presented in this book are excellent tools for enhancing muscle strength and size. However, even the best training procedures are only as productive as your ability to restore and rebuild sufficiently stressed muscle tissue to higher strength levels. There are three essential factors for maximizing muscle responsiveness—high-effort strength exercise, high-quality nutrition, and high-quantity rest.

In our opinion, high-intensity training is the most effective and efficient means for stimulating muscle and strength development. But, hard workouts represent only one side of the training triangle. For optimum muscle growth to occur, you must provide your body with a complete set of nutritional-building blocks. Even more importantly, you must allow ample recovery time between training sessions for protein resynthesis and muscle enlargement. Insufficient rest is undoubtedly the most prevalent problem preventing well-intentioned trainees from achieving their full strength potential.

All of the preceding chapters have dealt with high-intensity strength exercise, while this chapter addresses nutritional concerns and recovery recommendations for best training results.

Nutritional Considerations

While it is critically important to the strength-building process, high-intensity exercise is essentially a muscle stressor that causes tissue trauma. The point to remember is that, immediately following a high-intensity training session, your muscles are at a low functional level, and they must be restored nutritionally to gain strength and grow. A review of your need for an adequate intake of water, protein, and carbohydrates helps to explain why and how this restoration should occur.

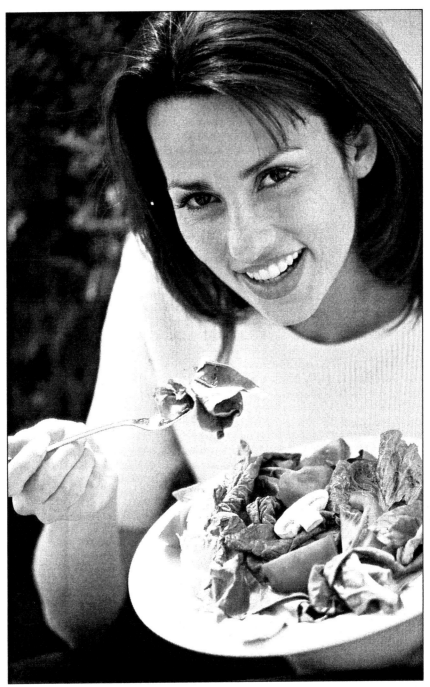

For optimal muscle growth to occur, you must provide your body with an adequate level of nutritional-building blocks.

• **Importance of Water**

The contractile components responsible for muscle movement are protein filaments, known as actin and myosin. However, protein does not represent the largest percentage of muscle tissue. By weight, muscle is approximately 25 percent protein and 75 percent water, making water the most important nutrient in a strength trainer's diet. Protein synthesis occurs in a fluid medium, and water is a major player in the muscle-building process. Trying to build muscle without adequate hydration is unwise and unsuccessful. Yet, many exercisers consume too little water to meet the physiological demands of high-intensity strength workouts.

Generally speaking, an individual who is engaged in strength exercise on an on-going basis needs about 50 percent more water than an inactive individual. Considering that the average adult is advised to drink eight glasses of water daily, regular strength exercisers should consume at least 12 glasses of fluids a day for optimum muscle development. It is recommended that at a minimum, you drink a glass of water before and after each strength workout, as well as whenever you feel the need to consume during your exercise session.

Although water is the preferred selection, other fluids may be substituted if you so desire. Alcoholic drinks and caffeinated beverages should be avoided because they have a diuretic effect. Fruit juices are superb sources of water, carbohydrates, and essential electrolytes, such as calcium, potassium and sodium. A 50-50 combination of soda water and fruit juice can provide a sparkling drink that has less sugar content than pure fruit juice. Low-fat milk is also an excellent fluid for strength trainers, because it provides water, protein and calcium necessary for muscle building.

• **Protein Requirements**

With respect to protein and calcium, all low-fat dairy items are ideal, including low-fat yogurt, low-fat cottage cheese, and even low-fat frozen yogurt. Other outstanding protein sources include egg whites, tuna fish, and turkey breast, although all seafood, poultry, and extra-lean cuts of meat are relatively high in protein and low in fat. Protein can also be obtained from several non-animal sources, such as wheat germ, whole grains, soy products, and various types of beans.

The general recommendation for protein intake is about one gram for every two pounds of bodyweight. However, people who perform high-intensity strength exercise may require up to twice as much protein, or one gram for every pound of bodyweight, for optimum muscle building.

For example, if you are a muscular 168 pounds, you may need as much as 168 grams of protein daily during high-intensity strength training periods. At 28 grams per ounce, this is equivalent to six ounces of protein per day. Because this amount of protein may be easily attained through normal dietary sources, it is not usually necessary to consume protein supplements. It is also unwise to eat excessive amounts of protein because the unused nitrogen component must be neutralized by calcium and excreted from the body, thereby reducing both calcium and water resources.

It is advisable to distribute your protein intake throughout the day to facilitate processing and tissue assimilation. Furthermore, some evidence exists that eating protein shortly after your strength training session may enhance the muscle-rebuilding process.

- **Carbohydrate Needs**

Because high-intensity exercise sessions require large amounts of energy, complex carbohydrates should comprise a significant percentage of the strength trainer's diet. The best sources of low-fat and high-nutrient carbohydrates are vegetables, fruits, whole-grain cereals and bread. Dried fruits, such as raisins and dates, are a fat-free alternative to cookies, candy bars and other sweets. Nuts, such as almonds, are a better crunchy choice than chips. Although somewhat high in fat, nuts are rich in both protein and many essential nutrients.

Generally speaking, the United States Department of Agriculture (USDA) Food Guide Pyramid offers a useful guideline to individuals who engage in strength exercise, with perhaps a little more emphasis in the meat and milk sections of the triangle for high-intensity strength trainers. The USDA 'Food Guide Pyramid recommends the following daily servings of six specific food categories:

#1.   Breads, cereals, pastries, grains . . . . .6-11 servings

#2.   Vegetables . . . . .3-5 servings

#3.   Fruits . . . . .2-4 servings

#4.   Milk, yogurt, cheese . . . . .2-3 servings

#5.   Meat, poultry, fish, eggs, nuts . . . . .2-3 servings

#6.   Fats, oils, sweets . . . . .Sparingly

We recommend that people who perform high-intensity strength exercise should consume extra servings of vegetables and fruits (including fruit juices) for high-energy workouts, and an extra serving or two of protein foods (low-fat dairy products and lean meats) for optimum muscle building.

Rest Recommendations

During the past several decades, people in modernized societies have been averaging less and less sleep on a daily basis. Many adults consider sleep a necessary evil that interferes with life. For some individuals, there never seem to be enough hours in the day to include a full night's repose. Certainly, the entertainment options offered by television and the excitement provided by the internet make it even more difficult to adhere to the old adage of "early to bed."

Recently research from leading universities has demonstrated that most Americans are attaining too little sleep to function at their best, physically or mentally. In fact, Americans are a severely sleep-deprived people who are typically restless during the night and listless during the day. Of course, both sides of this coin are equally important. You need to be more physically active during the day to sleep better during the night, and you need to sleep more during the night to function better during the day.

While it is true that some people need less sleep than others, the experts advise at least eight hours of daily sleep on average to support a fully functional lifestyle. In our experience, you should increase your standard sleep period by 30 to 60 minutes a night if you want to achieve the best results from your high-intensity strength training program. In other words, you should strive for eight and one-half to nine hours of sleep each night to maximize your strength gains and muscle development.

If this sounds like too much time spent sleeping, remember that well-rested individuals are far more productive than their chronically fatigued counterparts. All factors considered, you can accomplish tasks in less time and with fewer errors when you attain sufficient sleep. You should also discover that your strength exercises can be performed with more resistance when you have a full night's rest.

Keep in mind that an effective strength workout produces microtrauma in the muscle tissue, leaving it weaker than before the training session. It is only during the rest period that follows your workout that the stressed muscle tissue can be restored and restructured to higher levels of strength development. In a very real sense, the quantity of your rest is just as important as the quality of your training.

While it is very easy to sleep too little, it is unlikely that you will sleep too much. If you are not obtaining sufficient sleep, the alarm clock always appears to be an unwelcome intruder. However, when you are on an optimum sleeping schedule, you typically wake up on your own, feeling refreshed and ready for action. We therefore strongly suggest that you go to bed a little earlier when you perform high-intensity exercise in order to maximize your training investment. As simple as this seems, no single factor appears to be more closely related to the results of a high-effort strength training program.

High-Intensity Training Frequency

Sound sleep and quality rest can clearly enhance the effects of high-intensity strength training. However, due to the greater exercise effort and tissue trauma involved in high-intensity training, most people must reduce their workout frequency. The point to keep in mind is that high-intensity training sessions typically require longer recovery periods for maximum muscle building to occur.

Whereas, we normally recommend three standard total body workouts per week (Monday, Wednesday, Friday or Tuesday, Thursday, Saturday), high-intensity training sessions should be limited to twice a week. While we have experienced excellent results with a Monday and Friday exercise schedule, other two-day per week training frequencies should work equally well (e.g., Monday and Thursday, Tuesday and Friday, Wednesday and Saturday). More frequent high-intensity workouts typically lead to mental burnout and physical overtraining, both of which are counterproductive to strength gains and muscle development.

High-Intensity Training Duration

It has been aptly stated that you can train hard or you can train long, but you can't train hard for long. In other words, you may perform low-intensity strength exercise for a relatively long period of time, but you can perform high-intensity strength exercise for only a short period of time. It's almost like running. If you run at a moderate pace, you can run for a fairly long time period. However, if you sprint at a fast speed, you cannot continue for more than 30 to 90 seconds.

Each high-intensity exercise set is similar to sprinting, as you work at a near-maximum effort level until your anaerobic energy system fatigues (typically less than 90 seconds). Although different exercises address different muscle groups, the overall and cumulative physical exertion soon becomes evident. Consequently, few people can continue high-intensity strength training for more than 20 to 30 minutes per session.

We generally recommend between 10 and 16 exercises for each high-intensity strength training session. If you take up to 90 seconds per exercise and 20 seconds between exercises, each station requires less than two minutes. Therefore, you should complete a 10-exercise circuit in under 20 minutes and a 16-exercise circuit in about one-half hour. Training for longer periods of time can be challenging psychologically and demanding physiologically, but is unlikely to qualify as a really high-intensity exercise experience. For best results, you should strive to make each high-intensity strength training session hard in effort and relatively brief in duration.

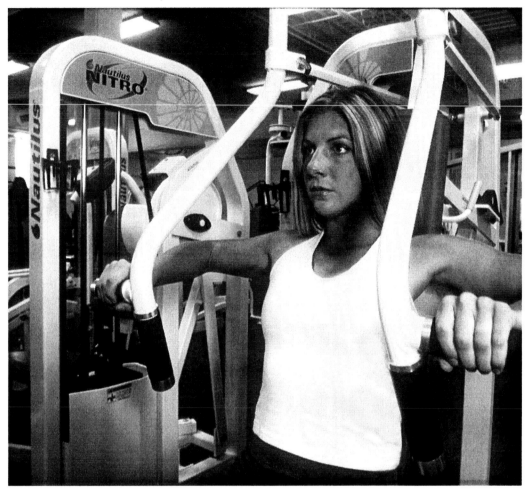

You can train hard or you can train long, but you can't train hard for long.

Concluding Comments

Proper nutrition, sound sleep, infrequent training sessions, and relatively brief workouts have been shown to enhance the effects of high-intensity strength exercise. In addition to adhering to the essential precepts inherent in a safe and sensible approach for increasing the strength-building stimulus, you should experience even better results by training with a competent instructor or partner. A watchful eye will reduce your chances of performing the exercises with poor technique, and an encouraging comment will help assure an honest effort from you on every training repetition and set.

Appendix:
Sample, Completed
Workout Cards

The workout cards presented in this Appendix illustrate actual training documents recorded for eight recent participants in our high-intensity strength training program. All of the exercisers completed our combined exercise protocol that included both the pre-exhaustion and assisted training techniques. Four people did the five-and-five protocol (five repetitions to fatigue, followed by five assisted repetitions) and four subjects did the eight-and-four protocol (eight repetitions to fatigue, followed by four assisted repetitions).

It should be noted that half of the participants were intermediate-level trainees (lower weightloads) and half were advanced-level trainees (higher weightloads). The key factor in each individual's weightload progression was reaching muscle fatigue at the prescribed number of repetitions. For example, if you are doing the eight-and-four protocol, you increase the resistance slightly when you complete nine repetitions in good form. Be sure that assisted repetitions are provided only when you reach muscle fatigue, and only on the lifting phase (concentric muscle action) of each post-fatigue repetition.

Needless to say, this type of high-intensity training works best in structured settings with strict exercise procedures and careful supervision. Emphasize proper exercise technique on every repetition and progress gradually as you gain strength. Two high-intensity training sessions per week should be sufficient for excellent results, because more demanding strength workouts require longer recovery periods for muscle-building processes to be completed.

In all likelihood, as you review the actual training progressions of these research subjects, you will gain a personal perspective on high-intensity strength training. You should note that the combined exercise protocol worked equally well for the four men and the four women, for the intermediate trainees and the advanced trainees, for the 23-year old and the 66-year old. You should observe that initial weightloads must sometimes be reduced to ensure proper and productive form (see Rich's leg-press progression). You should also see that different rates of progression were used in different exercises, such as Olivia's improvement in the leg extension (140 lbs to 215 lbs) and her improvement in the leg curl (140 lbs to 165 lbs). Most of all, we hope that you will find our participants' workout records educational and motivational for your own high-intensity training sessions.

NAME: <u>Sue</u>   AGE: <u>43</u>   GENDER: <u>Female</u>

WORKOUT DAYS: <u>Monday and Thursday</u>   TIME: <u>8:30 – 9:00 am</u>

PROTOCOL: 5 Repetitions to gatigue followed by 5 assisted reps.

FITNESS LEVEL: Intermediate

Workouts	1	2	3	4	5	6	7	8	9	10
Leg Extension	60	90	82.5	85	87.5	87.5	90	92.5	95	95
Leg Curl	60	70	72.5	75	77.5	77.5	77.5	80	82.5	85
Leg Press	120	135	165	175	175	170	175	175	185	195
Chest Cross	55	60	62.5	65	67.5	70	72.5	70	70	70
Chest Press	55	70	72.5	75	75	75	77.5	77.5	80	80
Pullover	60	65	67.5	70	72.5	72.5	75	75	77.5	80
Compound Row	70	73	80	85	90		92	94	97	102
Lateral Raise	55	55	57.5	60	62.5	62.5	65	65	67.5	70
Overhead Press	40	50	45	47	49	55	57	57	59	61
Biceps Curl	50	555	7.5	60	65	65	65	65	67.5	70
Triceps Extension	50	45	45	47.5	47.5	47.5	50	50	52.5	52.5
Abdominal	60	60	60	60	60	62.5	62.5	62.5	62.5	62.5

	Before High Intensity Training	**After High Intensity Training**
Chin-ups	5	10
Dips	9	15

NAME: <u>Chris</u>   AGE: <u>36</u>   GENDER: <u>Male</u>

WORKOUTDAYS: <u>TuesdayandFriday</u>   TIME: <u>9:30–10:00am</u>

PROTOCOL: 5 Repetitions to fatigue followed by 5 assisted reps.

FITNESSLEVEL: Intermediate

Workouts	1	2	3	4	5	6	7	8	9	10
Leg Extension	120	122.5	125	127.5	130	132.5	135	140	145	150
Leg Curl	100	102.5	105	107.5	110	115	117.5	122.5	125	130
Leg Press	260	270	275	280	285	290	295	300	305	310
Chest Cross	90	92.5	95	97.5	100	102.5	105	107.5	110	112.5
Chest Press	100	102.5	105	107.5	110	115	117.5	120	122.5	125
Pullover	110	112.5	115	117.5	120	125	127.5	130	132.5	135
Compound Row	100	105	110	112	115	117	120	123	125	130
Lateral Raise	65	67.5	70	72.5	75	77.5	80	82.5	85	90
Overhead Press	55	65	67	70	72	74	76	78	80	82
Biceps Curl	60	70	72.5	75	77.5	80	82.5	85	87.5	90
Triceps Extension	55	60	62.5	65	67.5	70	72.5	75	77.5	80
Abdominal	100	102.5	105	107.5	110	112.5	115	117.5	120	120

	Before High Intensity Training	**After High Intensity Training**
Chin-ups	1	2
Dips	1	3

NAME: Olivia   AGE: 23   GENDER: Female

WORK OUT DAYS: Monday and Friday   TIME: 11–11:30am

PROTOCOL: 5 Repetitions to fatigue followed by 5 assisted reps.

FITNESS LEVEL: Advanced

Workouts	1	2	3	4	5	6	7	8	9	10
Leg Extension	140	155	165	175	180	190	200	205	210	215
Leg Curl	140	142	144	147	150	155	157	160	162	165
Leg Press	250	275	277.5	280	282.5	285	290	295	300	305
Chest Cross	90	90	90	92.5	92.5	95	97.5	100	102.5	105
Chest Press	125	125	127.5	130	130	132.5	135	137.5	140	145
Pullover	100	102.5	105	107.5	110	112	115	117.5	120	122.5
Compound Row	135	140	145	147	149	150	152	154	156	158
Lateral Raise	90	92.5	95	97.5	100	102.5	105	107.5	110	112.5
Overhead Press	90	90	92	92	95	95	97	97	100	102.5
Biceps Curl	70	72.5	75	77.5	80	82.5	85	87.5	90	92.5
Triceps Extension	60	62.5	65	67.5	70	72.5	75	77.5	80	82.5
Abdominal	100	105	110	115	120	125	130	135	140	142.5

	Before High Intensity Training	After High Intensity Training
Chin-ups	**4**	**9**
Dips	**24**	**30**

NAME: <u>William</u>   AGE: <u>40</u>   GENDER: <u>Male</u>

WORK OUT DAYS: <u>Monday and Thursday</u>   TIME: <u>8–8:30am</u>

PROTOCOL: 5 Repetitions to fatigue followed by 5 assisted reps.

FITNESS LEVEL: Advanced

Workouts	1	2	3	4	5	6	7	8	9	10
Leg Extension	150	170	200	230	240	255	265	270	270	275
Leg Curl	120	125	128	140	140	143	143	143	145	147
Chest Cross	150	170	170	180	182.5	185	187.5	187.5	185	187.5
Chest Press	200	220	240	245	247.5	250	252.5	257.5	260	265
Pullover	160	180	185	190	192.5	195	195	197.5	200	200
Compound Row	190	220	232	245	245	248	250	255	255	258
Lateral Raise	120	125	135	145	155	157	160	165	170	170
Overhead Press	180	180	185	188	190	190	195	198	200	200
Biceps Curl	135	137.5	135	135	137.5	137.5	140	145	145	145
Triceps Extension	110	125	127.5	135	135	135	137.5	140	145	145
Abdominal	100	90	100	115	120	125	125	127.5	130	130

	Before High Intensity Training	**After High Intensity Training**
Chin-ups	15	16
Dips	20	26

NAME: <u>Shauna</u>   AGE: <u>26</u>   GENDER: <u>Female</u>

WORK OUT DAYS: <u>Tuesday and Friday</u>   TIME: <u>8—8:30am</u>

PROTOCOL: 8 Repetitions to fatigue followed by 4 assisted reps.

FITNESS LEVEL: Intermediate

Workout	1	2	3	4	5	6	7	8	9	10
Leg Extension	70	75	77	80	85	87	92	97.5	102	110
Leg Curl	50	55	57	60	62	65	67	70	75	80
Leg Press	160	165	167	170	170	170	172	185	190	195
Chest Cross	40	45	47	50	52	55	57	60	60	60
Chest Press	55	57	60	62	65	67	70	70	72	75
Pullover	60	62	65	67	70	72	75	80	80	82
Torso Arm	65	67	70	72	75	77	80	85	87	90
Lateral Raise	40	42	45	45	45	45	47	47	47	47
Overhead Press	30	30	32	32	32	32	35	35	37	37
Biceps Curl	30	35	37	40	40	40	42	42	45	45
Triceps Extension	25	30	32	32	35	37	40	42	42	45
Abdominal	55	55	57	57	60	62	65	67	70	72

	Before High Intensity Training	**After High Intensity Training**
Chin-ups	0	1 (almost)
Dips	0	5

NAME: Peg   AGE: 66   GENDER: Female

WORK OUT DAYS: Monday and Friday   TIME: 10–10:30am

PROTOCOL: 8 Repetitions to fatigue followed by 4 assisted reps.

FITNESS LEVEL: Intermediate

Workouts	1	2	3	4	5	6	7	8	9	10
Leg Extension	120	125	130	135	135	135	140	145	147.5	150
Leg Curl	65	65		65	70	70	70	72.5	72.5	72.5
Leg Press	170	170	170	175	180	185	185	187.5	190	200
Chest Cross	60	60	60	65	65	65	65	67.5	70	72.5
Chest Press	65	65	65	70	70	70	70	70	70	70
Pullover	50	60	65	70	70	75	75	75	77.5	80
Torso Arm	50	60	70	75	75	80	80	82.5	82.5	85
Lateral Raise	35	40	40	42.5	42.5	42.5	42.5	42.5	42.5	42.5
Overhead Press	30	30	25	27.5	27.5	30	30	30	30	30
Biceps Curl	30	35	40	40	40	40	40	40	40	42.5
Triceps Extension	30	35	40	40	40	40	42.5	42.5	45	47.5
Abdominal	50	55	55	57.5	57.5	60	65	70	70	72.5

	Before High Intensity Training	**After High Intensity Training**
Chin-ups	0	1 (almost)
Dips	2	8

NAME: <u>Dick</u>   AGE: <u>49</u>   GENDER: <u>Male</u>

WORK OUT DAYS: <u>Tuesday and Friday</u>   TIME: <u>11:30—Noon</u>

PROTOCOL: 8 Repetitions to fatigue followed by 4 assisted reps.

FITNESS LEVEL: Advanced

Workouts	1	2	3	4	5	6	7	8	9	10
Leg Extension	200	202.5	205	207.5	207.5	210	215	217.5	220	222.5
Leg Curl	110	112.5	115	117.5	117.5	120	122.5	125	127.5	130
Leg Press	360	362.5	365	367.5	367.5	370	375	379.5	380	385
Chest Cross	140	142.5	145	147.5	150	152.5	155	157.5	160	162.5
Chest Press	155	157.5	160	162.5	165	167.5	170	172.5	175	197.5
Pullover	175	177.5	180	182.5	185	187.5	190	192.5	195	197.5
Torso Arm	170	172.5	175	177.5	180	182.5	185	187.5	190	192.5
Lateral Raise	95	97.5	100	102.5	105	107.5	110	112.5	115	117.5
Overhead Press	100	102.5	105	107.5	110	112.5	115	117.5	117.5	120
Biceps Curl	95	97.5	100	102.5	105	107.5	107.5	105	105	107.5
Triceps Extension	85	87.5	90	92.5	95	97.5	100	100	100	102.5
Abdominal	140	142.5	145	147.5	150	152.5	155	160	162.5	165

	Before High Intensity Training	**After High Intensity Training**
Chin-ups	11	14
Dips	14	15

NAME: <u>Rich</u>   AGE: <u>36</u>   GENDER: <u>Male</u>

WORK OUT DAYS: <u>Monday and Friday</u>   TIME: <u>9:30–10:30am</u>

PROTOCOL: 8 Repetitions to fatigue followed by 4 assisted reps.

FITNESS LEVEL: Advanced

Workouts	1	2	3	4	5	6	7	8	9	10
Leg Extension	190	190	195	200	205	210	215	220	225	230
Leg Curl	105	105	110	115	120	120	122.5	125	125	127.5
Leg Press	400	385	390	395	395	395	400	405	410	415
Chest Cross	165	165	170	175	180	185	187.5	190	192.5	195
Chest Press	165	165	170	172.5	172.5	175	175	175	175	177.5
Pullover	220	220	225	230	235	240	242.5	242.5	242.5	245
Torso Arm	160	160	165	170	175	177.5	177.5	200	200	200
Lateral Raise	115	115	120	125	127.5	130	130	132.5	135	140
Overhead Press	100	105	110	115	117.5	120	130	132.5	135	135
Biceps Curl	85	85	90	90	92.5	95	100	102.5	105	107.5
Triceps Extension	145	145	145	145	147.5	150	150	150	150	155
Abdominal	165	165	170	175	177.5	180	180	182.5	185	187.5

	Before High Intensity Training	**After High Intensity Training**
Chin-ups	6	8
Dips	15	18

About the Authors

Wayne L. Westcott, Ph.D., is Fitness Research Director at the South Shore YMCA in Quincy, Massachusetts, where he conducts studies on strength training with youth, adults and seniors, as well as special populations. Dr. Westcott has authored more than a dozen books on strength training, and has written hundreds of articles related to resistance exercise and physical fitness. He has also lectured extensively throughout the United States, Canada, and Europe on sensible strength exercise. Dr. Westcott has served as a fitness advisor to the President's Council on Physical Fitness and Sports, the YMCA of the USA, the Governor's Committee on Physical Fitness and Sports, the International Association of Fitness Professionals, the American Council on Exercise, the American Senior Fitness Association, the National Youth Sports Safety Foundation, and the National Strength Professionals Association. He has also served on the editorial board for numerous publications, including *Shape, Fitness, Prevention, Men's Health, Club Industry, American Fitness Quarterly*, and *Nautilus Magazine*. His contributions to the field of fitness have been widely recognized, as evidenced by the following professional honors: Lifetime Achievement Award from the International Association of Fitness Professionals; Healthy American Fitness Leader Award from the President's Council on Physical Fitness and Sports; Lifetime Achievement Award from the Governor's Committee on Physical Fitness and Sports; Roberts-Gulick Memorial Award from the YMCA Association of Professional Directors; and NOVA 7 Award for Program Excellence from Fitness Management Magazine. Dr. Westcott and his wife, Claudia, reside in Abington, Massachusetts.

Tracy D'Arpino holds a B.S. in health and fitness and is a licensed physical therapy assistant. She is the Associate Fitness Research Director at the South Shore YMCA, where she has conducted several research studies with Dr. Westcott on high-intensity strength training. In addition to her work with advanced strength training techniques, Tracy has developed numerous fitness programs for people with disabilities. These include the "Partnership Program" for quadriplegics, stroke victims, blind, deaf and other physically challenged individuals, the "Conquer Life Program" for cancer patients, the "Kids in Motion Program" for children with special needs and the "Focus on Abilities Program" for emotionally challenged adults. Tracy has worked closely with Wayne for almost 10 years, and together they have done several high-intensity strength training workshops for the fitness instructors in the United States Navy. Tracy, who lives in Quincy, MA, is an avid marathon runner, triathlete, and fitness enthusiast.